aakp

American Association of Kidney Patients

AAKP Programs

AT HOME with aakp

aakp **RENALIFE**

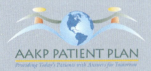
AAKP PATIENT PLAN
Providing Today's Patients with Answers for Tomorrow

aakp **HealthLine**
Listen. Learn. Live.

My Health™

The American Association of Kidney Patients is a national organization directed by kidney patients for kidney patients.

For more than 40 years, AAKP has been dedicated to providing education and support to kidney patients, their family members and renal professionals through a variety of activities including:

- Assisting patients both to learn more about their disease and to become active participants in planning and managing their treatment;

- Improving patient understanding of and access to rehabilitation;

- Working together for the improvement of public programs that help kidney patients meet their health care and personal needs;

- Reflecting the views and concerns of patients to public policy makers and others in the renal community;

- And providing a lifeline for patients in need of emotional support and reassurance that only other patients can provide.

aakp
The voice of all kidney patients™

**2701 North Rocky Point Drive, Suite 150
Tampa, Florida 33607
800-749-2257
www.aakp.org**

Want more information on AAKP programs?

Name _____

Mailing Address _____

City _____ State _____ Zipcode _____

Telephone _____

Email address _____

Please let us know if you are a: ☐ patient ☐ family member ☐ health care professional ☐ physician

☐ *chronic kidney disease (CKD)* ☐ *dialysis* ☐ *transplant recipient*

American Kidney Fund®

reaching out | giving hope | improving lives

The mission of the American Kidney Fund is to fight kidney disease through direct financial support to patients in need; health education; and prevention efforts. The American Kidney Fund leads the nation in providing charitable assistance to dialysis patients who need help with the costs associated with treating kidney failure. In 2010, 101,000 people—1 out of every 4 dialysis patients in the United States—received assistance from the American Kidney Fund for health insurance premiums and other treatment-related expenses. Millions of people nationwide benefit annually from the American Kidney Fund's efforts to fight kidney disease through health education and prevention efforts. The American Kidney Fund's national campaign, *Pair Up: Join the Fight to Prevent Kidney Disease*, empowers women to protect themselves—and the people they love—from kidney disease. The American Kidney Fund offers free kidney health screenings in communities nationwide, as well as extensive online health education materials and courses and a toll-free health information **HelpLine (866.300.2900).**

As a nine-time recipient of the top "Four Star" rating from Charity Navigator, the American Kidney Fund is ranked among the top 1 percent of charities nationwide for fiscal accountability. In addition, the American Kidney Fund holds an A+ rating from the American Institute of Philanthropy; adheres to the National Health Council Standards of Excellence; and is a member of the Better Business Bureau Wise Giving Alliance.

For More Information

▶ Visit our website **KidneyFund.org**

▶ Call our HelpLine **866.300.2900**

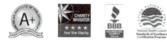

Help, I Need Dialysis!

How to have a good future with kidney disease

Dori Schatell, MS | *John Agar, MD*

The authors extend our profound gratitude to the people with kidney disease and the clinicians who took the time to review this book draft and provide their comments. Each of your contributions helped to create a better final product, an d we appreciate your time and thoughtfulness more than we can say. We are also very grateful for a generous donation that made possible all of the original illustrations in this book and helped bring the concepts to life.

Disclaimer

Help, I Need Dialysis! is a guide for people who have chronic kidney disease or kidney failure. Use of this book does not replace the need to talk with your doctor and healthcare team about your care and your options. If medical advice or other expert help is needed, seek the advice of a competent professional.

A book such as this one can only draw from the information on hand as of the date of publication. While the authors have made every effort to assure that the contents of the book are accurate and complete, no guarantees can be given. The Medical Education Institute, Inc., authors, and advertisers are not responsible for errors or omissions or for any consequences from use of the contents of this book and make no warranty, expressed or implied, with respect to the currency, completeness, or accuracy of the contents of the publication. Future medical advances, product updates, or changes to the law may affect or change the information in this book. Neither the Medical Education Institute, Inc. nor the authors are under any obligation to update the contents of *Help, I Need Dialysis!*

To the extent permitted by law, the authors and the Medical Education Institute, Inc. disclaim all liability for any damages or injury caused by any error, omission, deletion, defect, access to, alteration of, or use of *Help, I Need Dialysis!* The contents of *Help, I Need Dialysis!*, including, but not limited to text, graphics, and icons, are trademarked materials owned or controlled by the Medical Education Institute, Inc.

Help, I Need Dialysis!

How to have a good future with kidney disease

A Book for People with Stage 3–5 CKD

Each year, more than 100,000 Americans start dialysis. Complete, accurate information about ALL dialysis options has been hard to find…until now.

Anyone facing the life-changing decisions that come with kidney failure simply must read ***Help! I Need Dialysis.*** *This information could add years and quality to their lives.*

About the authors. Two credible, renowned authors who are passionate about better treatments have collaborated on this book. Together they tell the full story.

Dori Schatell, MS — Executive Director of the non-profit Medical Education Institute. Ms. Schatell has 23 years of experience specializing in evidence-based and empowering patient education. She has written hundreds of educational pieces, conducted research and published peer-reviewed articles in nephrology, and launched several award-winning websites including Kidney School and Home Dialysis Central.

John Agar, MD — Emeritus Director of Nephrology and Chief of Service (Medicine) at Barwon Health in Geelong, Australia. Areas of interest include extended-hour and frequency hemo-dialysis, and optimal dialysis. He is Clinical Associate Professor of Medicine, University of Melbourne, has published widely, and runs the popular site: NocturnalDialysis.org.

About the Medical Education Institute, Inc.

The non-profit Medical Education Institute, which was founded in 1992, serves the mission of helping people with chronic disease learn to manage and improve their health. Our vision is to create a world where people with chronic kidney disease are knowledgeable, active partners in their medical care, using treatment options that allow them to live full, productive lives. Our programs include Kidney School (**www.kidneyschool.org**), Home Dialysis Central (**www.homedialysis.org**), and Life Options (**www.lifeoptions.org**). Our support comes from educational grants, government contracts, project fees, sponsorships from corporations, and individual donations.

Foreword

"Knowledge is an antidote to fear" Ralph Waldo Emerson

Being diagnosed with chronic kidney disease and needing dialysis is scary. You are undoubtedly afraid and probably feel totally overwhelmed. You have dozens of questions, but may not know where to find answers. Most of all, you wonder if life will ever be the same again.

Although life on dialysis may be different, it can still be very, very good. This book will help you fit dialysis into your lifestyle and live life on your own terms. It will arm you with the knowledge you need to understand the many different facets of dialysis care and to maintain your quality of life.

Knowledge is power—the power to make the best choices, to take control of your health, and to be an equal partner on your health team. After all, we are a society of "take charge" people. We love to be the one to "call the shots." Yet we are often hesitant to transfer that assertive "can-do" attitude to the seemingly mysterious area of health care. The contents of this book will help you and your care partner do just that.

That's not to minimize the adjustments. Anything new can be daunting. Think about learning to drive as a teenager. You might have been nervous about negotiating traffic and worried about fender benders, but by taking it "step by step" you became a confident, competent driver. Believe me; it's not any different with dialysis!

Will there be bumps in the road? Absolutely. Will it always be easy? Of course not. However, consider this simple truism: most things in life are not without their unique challenges. I assure you that your life can be as good and as fulfilling as before, maybe even more so!

You may be thinking "who is she to tell us that a good life can coexist with dialysis"? I do speak from a certain amount of experience—besides being a nurse, my late husband was on home hemodialysis for 25 years. During the entire time, he worked 50-60 hours per week, played golf, and volunteered in our community. Together we traveled, renovated an old house and raised our son. You too can still have a busy, satisfying life.

The authors begin with the basics and gradually strip away the complexities of dialysis by presenting concepts in a straightforward, understandable way. The book is divided into easily readable chapters, each on a specific aspect of dialysis in a stand alone format for quick reference. Topics run the entire gamut from the role of the kidneys to the process of dialysis to questions about intimacy…and everything in between. Interspersed in the chapters are stories of real people on dialysis, those whose lives are immensely rewarding and personally satisfying.

Ms. Schatell and Dr. Agar bring literally decades of experience and expertise in the kidney community to the writing of this excellent book. Both authors are so in tune with those on dialysis that I have often accused them of being "patients in disguise."

A final cautionary word: Being on dialysis won't automatically elevate you or your care partner to a state of instant perfection. You carry your former self into this new chapter of your life. You are the same person with the same hopes, dreams and goals as before and being able to pursue those goals is as important now as it ever was. This book will help you do that.

The authors say it best: this book's goal is "to demystify kidneys and dialysis and to help you take charge of your health care." They have succeeded admirably.

Denise Eilers, RN, BSN

Table of Contents

Become Your Own Expert

KEY POINT

You have options. You can match your treatment choice to your lifestyle. Learn all you can so you can choose a treatment that will help you feel your best and live your life the way you want to.

There are 305 million people in the U.S., and about one in 12 have some degree of chronic kidney disease (CKD).[1] More than half a million are being treated for kidney failure right now with dialysis and transplant. And each year, more than 100,000 people learn that their kidneys have failed. *You are not alone.*

You may not have known it was happening, but kidney failure from CKD is a long, slow process that takes months or years. Each kidney has about a million *nephrons* to filter the blood. You can lose most of your kidney function before you notice any symptoms. Some people say they feel fine and can't believe their kidneys don't work, even when blood tests show the damage.

Learning that you will need dialysis or a kidney transplant is a shock for you and the people who care about you. Maybe the news was a bolt from the blue, and you just found out. Or, maybe you're on dialysis now and want to know how your treatment works and how you can feel your best. Either way, we wrote this book for you. We're on your side. Here, you can learn what you need to know to make choices that can help you live a good life.

A *good* life? With *dialysis*? Is that even possible?

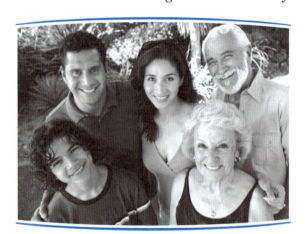

Yes. Kidney failure is the end of your kidneys—but it does *not* have to be the end of you, and your goals and dreams. If you make good choices, you may feel well and have enough energy to finish school, keep your job, do Ironman triathlons, go kayaking, climb a mountain, or ride a bike across the U.S. We are not making this up: people on dialysis have done *every one* of these things. Of course, not everyone on dialysis climbs mountains! Chances are, the folks who do so started before their kidneys failed. But if you have a passion—from baking to square dancing, or from working in your garden to raising prize puppies— dialysis alone should not stop you from doing it.

As Douglas Adams says in the *Hitchhiker's Guide to the Galaxy*, "Don't panic." You have options. Many other health problems don't have effective treatments. Just 40 years ago, there were not enough dialysis machines to help all of those who had kidney failure. The treatment was experimental and costly. Most health plans would not pay for it. In some parts of the U.S., like Seattle, "Life or Death" committees of citizens and clergy would decide who would get the treatment and live—and who would not.[2] Today, some people live fully for decades with dialysis and/or kidney transplant(s), and you'll meet some of them in these pages. In the past, most were not so fortunate. It may not seem like it right now, but in a very real way, you are lucky.

A Normal Life

Your goal is to have as normal a life as you can despite your kidney failure, isn't it?

- You want to feel good from one day to the next.
- You want to keep your job if you have one, and your health plan.
- You want to spend time with your family and friends and be able to plan ahead.
- You want to keep doing your hobbies or volunteer work.
- You may be in a relationship—or want one—that includes a loving sex life, and want that to continue. Depending on your age, you may want to have a child.
- You want to eat good food, and not have to worry too much about what is or isn't in it to keep you healthy.
- You want a nice cool iced tea or lemonade on a hot day.
- You don't want to take (and pay for) a dozen or more pills each day.
- You don't want to be a burden on your loved ones.
- You don't want to have to think about kidney disease day in and day out.

We can help. Our goal is to help you become your own expert so you can reach your goals.

Your Job in Your Kidney Disease

This book will demystify kidneys and dialysis and help you take charge of your health care. That may sound a bit strange, since we're used to thinking doctors are in charge. And, if you have a sudden, curable "acute" health problem, like a broken arm, that makes sense. You are in pain; the doctor can fix you. You get a cast put on, rest and take pain pills, and in a few weeks you're better.

Chronic, long-term health problems like kidney disease are not the same as an acute illness. You have to deal with your illness all day long, day in and day out. But you may only see your doctor once a month for a few minutes. Even if you are on dialysis now, three times a week, your treatment is only supervised for about 14 hours a week—out of 168. That's just 8% of your time. Yet in the 92% of the time that you're out in the world on your own, *you* decide what to eat and drink, manage your symptoms, take prescribed drugs (or not), and advocate for yourself. All of that is part of what we call *self-management*.

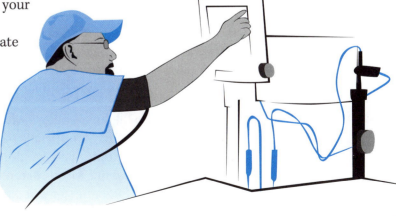

We don't call you a "patient" in this book. Do you have an illness? Yes. But whether you want it or not, chronic disease gives you a new job: to keep a positive attitude, learn all you can, and take an active role in your care—not a *patient* one. Your job is to self-manage. In other words, you need to become your own expert. So, in our book, you're a person who self-manages a chronic disease, not a patient.

How do we know that becoming your own expert is important? We talked to people who lived on hemodialysis for 15 years or more. We do research with people who have kidney disease. We've talked to *thousands* of people over the years who have kidney disease and asked what helps them most, in person, on the phone, and through email. You can see our other efforts to educate people about kidney disease and kidney failure on our websites:

www.homedialysis.org | www.kidneyschool.org
www.lifeoptions.org | www.nocturnaldialysis.org

You Have Choices

Most people who face dialysis don't know that their choice of treatment will affect *every* aspect of their lives. In 2009, 91.7% of people on dialysis in the U.S., did hemodialysis (HD) in a clinic three times a week, for 3–4 hours at a time.[3] We call this "standard in-center HD." Most of those 91.7% never even knew they had other options. In fact, the only large study of options awareness in the U.S. found that just 1 in 4 knew of any treatment other than standard HD.[4]

In 2008, Medicare changed the rules for dialysis clinics. Now clinics are *required* to tell you about ALL of the treatment options for kidney failure *and* where to get them. This book may help them do that.

When you finish this book, you will know how your treatment choice can affect:

- **What you can eat and drink**
- **How many drugs you need to take**
- **How much energy you will have**
- **How well you will sleep**
- **Your sex life and whether you can carry or father children**
- **Whether you will be able to keep your job (and health plan)**
- **How often you will be in the hospital**
- **How long you may live**

We'll tell you all about it. We've used hundreds of references from medical journals so you have proof that can help you talk with your doctor about what you want to do. And, we share stories from real people who have faced the same choices you face now, so you can see how things are working out for them.

Something else that many people with kidney failure don't know is that *you can change treatments*. (NOTE: Some people call treatment options "modalities.") If one treatment fit everyone all the time, there wouldn't be a need for all of the other options. Based on what you want *your* life to look like, one treatment may be a better fit for you now. Another may work out better for you down the road. Or, you may try a treatment that sounds like a perfect fit, but doesn't work out that way. That's okay, you can switch. In a long life with kidney failure, it's likely that you'll use more than one type of treatment. That's not a failure, it's a life plan!

Try Treatments on for Size

A long-time kidney disease educator has some good advice about choosing a treatment. She suggests that you think through your day and how it might work with each type of treatment you are thinking about:[5]

- **Wake up** – What time would you want to get up? To start or stop treatment for the day? Do you mind seeing dialysis equipment or supplies in your home, or would this be a deal-breaker for you? Do you want to be able to choose when to wake up, or is it okay if a clinic tells you to arrive at 5:00 a.m.?

- **Eat breakfast** – What sort of diet and fluid limits are you willing to live with each day? Standard in-center HD has the most limits, peritoneal dialysis (PD) and short daily HD have fewer, nocturnal HD has the least.

- **Take medications** – How many pills will you want to take in a day? Standard in-center HD has the most pills (about half of people who use it need to take 19 pills a day). Nocturnal HD has the least.

- **Go to work** – Do you have a job? How will your treatment times fit your work life, and how much control will you have? How much will your income drop if you quit your job and take disability? Social Security Disability takes 6 months to start, and pays only about 35% of the average worker's earned income.

- **Get your treatments** – If you live far from a clinic or don't have a car, in-center HD can be costly and inconvenient. Home treatments mean that after training you visit the clinic just once or twice a month for clinic appointments. PD or short daily HD treatments can be done throughout the day—is that a plus or a minus for you?

- **Deal with childcare** – Do you have young or school-aged children? Who will care for them if you get your treatments in a clinic? What will happen during school vacations or summer breaks?

- **Eat dinner** – How much will family meals be affected by your diet limits? Will your treatment give you the energy to cook? If not, who will prepare meals?

- **Spend time with family and friends** – Headaches, muscle cramps, and fatigue can keep you from making plans and having fun with your loved ones. What's important to you?

- **Go to bed** – How well are you sleeping on your treatment choice? Could you sleep with a machine in the room? Could you sleep in a clinic for nocturnal treatments? How will your body image and sex life be affected by your treatment choice?

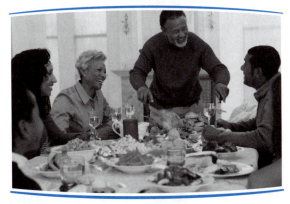

There are no right or wrong answers to any of these questions—only what will or won't work for *you*. Your needs may change over time, too. People who have lived with kidney failure for decades often find that over the years they may try *all* of the dialysis types, plus one or more transplants. We will freely admit our bias up front, though: if you use dialysis, *more is better* for both your short- and long-term health.

Every treatment for kidney disease has pros and cons. You are the only one who can decide what will best fit your needs and your lifestyle at any given time. We hope you'll choose a form of dialysis that is more like having healthy kidneys and will help you to feel your best and do what's most important to you. If you choose standard in-center HD, we'll tell you how to get the most benefit from it.

Once you make a choice, you need a *nephrologist* (kidney doctor) who will support you and prescribe it. Your treatment choice affects your lifestyle and even how long you may live. Making a treatment choice for yourself is key to how well you may do. One large study put 2,418 people new to dialysis into three groups, based on how they chose a treatment:[6]

- Group 1 (636 people) made their own choice
- Group 2 (922 people) worked with their care team to decide
- Group 3 (860 people) said their care team chose for them

Five years later, those who made their *own* choice (Group 1) *were significantly more likely to live longer and to get a transplant.* This was true even after adjusting for age, sex, race, other illness, blood test levels, level of kidney function, education, work, and marital status.

You are the one who must live with the treatment from day to day. It makes sense that you'll feel better if the choice is yours. This may mean that you have to persuade your doctor—or change doctors.

By the way, you don't have to read this book cover to cover. Jump around! Look for what you need right now. If you find that a section has too much detail for you now, skip past it. You can always choose to go back later and delve deeper if you want to.

What Treatment Would Kidney Doctors Choose for Themselves?

In 2010, the Medical Education Institute did a national survey of U.S. nephrologists to find out what they thought about dialysis.[7] One question we asked was, *"If you had kidney failure and had to wait 5 years for a transplant, which type of dialysis would you choose?"* See the pie chart for what the 629 respondents said.

So, all told, 94% of nephrologists would choose an option *other than* standard in-center HD—yet nearly all Americans with kidney failure get this option. Why? Good question. We suspect there may be a few reasons:

- They're doctors – they figure they can learn the treatment, but you can't (prove them wrong!).
- They don't trust that people who go home for dialysis will really do their treatments.
- It's easier for doctors to have folks dialyze in clinics, where they can see lots of people all at once.

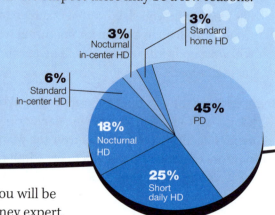

Read on! By the time you finish this book, you will be well on your way to becoming your own kidney expert.

Coping with Crisis

There is no question that kidney failure is a blow. Perhaps it is one that you knew was coming, or perhaps it came as the most unwelcome of surprises. Victor Frankl, an Austrian doctor, spent 3 years in a concentration camp during the Holocaust. Of his whole family, only he and one sister lived. Dr. Frankl is best known for being able to find meaning in even the worst of events. He said, "*The one thing you can't take away from me is the way I choose to respond to what you do to me. The last of one's freedoms is to choose one's attitude in any given circumstance*." This is true for you, too. You can't always choose what happens to you, but you *always* have a choice about how you deal with it.

An Old Chinese Story

There is always more than one way to look at something. This tale may help you see that the same event may be good—or bad:

A farmer had just one horse, and one day the horse ran away. The neighbors came to console him for his loss. "*This is awful!*" they said. The farmer said, "*What makes you think this is so bad?*"

The next month, the horse came home—with two wild horses. The farmer's neighbors were thrilled at his good luck. "*Such lovely strong horses!*" The farmer said, "*What makes you think this is so good?*"

The farmer's son was thrown from one of the wild horses and broke his leg. All the neighbors were sad. "*Such bad luck!*" The farmer said, "*What makes you think this is so bad?*" he asked...

A war came, and all of the able-bodied men were sent into battle. The farmer's son remained home, because of his broken leg. The neighbors were happy for the farmer. "*What makes you think this is good?*" he asked...

A life event like kidney failure does not have to be all bad:

- It can help you learn more about yourself and the people around you.

- It can help you sort out the *real* priorities in your life from the things that take up your time for no good reason.

- It can help you choose goals for what you want to achieve and help you find new ways of doing things.

- Having kidney failure can help you appreciate some of the everyday little things that you might otherwise ignore.

- You will meet new people who may prove to be important to you.

Would you choose kidney failure if the decision were up to you? We doubt it. But you can still find things to value out of the experience.

You Have Coped Before

You have likely lived through some other crisis in your life before now. Loss of a loved one, a job, a home. Another illness. A car crash. Think about what helped you then: support from others, learning what to expect (the unknown is much more frightening than the known), setting small goals, giving yourself time. Talking to people can help—and talking to people who know what you are going through may be the most helpful of all. With kidney failure, it may be a challenge to find someone who knows how to help. Voluntary kidney organizations (check Chapter 14 of this book for a list), peer-to-peer or "buddy" programs, or the social worker at the dialysis clinic are good places to start. For more general support, your religious advisor or a therapist may be able to offer some comfort and advice as to how to move forward.

You may have a number of conflicting emotions. It is very normal to be sad, afraid, angry—or all three at once—when you find out your body has let you down. Maybe you feel guilty, as if it is your fault your kidneys failed, because you did not take your doctor's advice. Or, perhaps your doctor missed your problem until it was too late, and you are furious. We have even met people who feel "unclean" because their kidneys don't work, and ashamed to tell others because they feel like pariahs. If you have heard of Dr. Elisabeth Kubler-Ross, you may recall that in her research, she found five stages of grief:

- **Denial** – *this is just not happening.*
- **Anger** – *it's not fair!*
- **Bargaining** – *if this goes away, I'll never smoke cigarettes again...*
- **Depression** – *what's the point?*
- **Acceptance** – *it's going to be okay; I'll find a way to make this work.*

You truly are grieving for the loss of yourself as a "healthy" person, or at least a person who doesn't have kidney failure. Losses can take time and support to come to terms with. And once you think you have done so, a health setback can send you through the stages all over again. People may not go through all of the stages or go through them in this order. This is normal! You are in the process of becoming a new person. You may have some bad days, 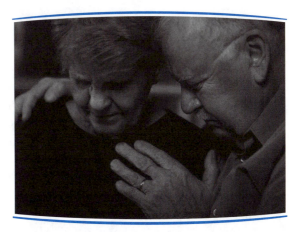 or "pity parties." But if you find that you aren't having *any* good days, or you have far more bad days than good ones, you'll want to make some changes.

Our brief, multiple choice quiz can help you look at your own attitude. There are no right or wrong answers, just circle the ones that best fit you. Give it a try:

Kidney Attitude Quiz

1. Why do you think kidney disease happened to you?

A. It was what I needed to have happen
B. Because of my mistakes
C. Random chance
D. I seem to attract troubles often
E. Nothing ever goes right for me

2. What have you learned from having kidney disease?

A. How to turn lemons into lemonade
B. How to overcome obstacles
C. Nothing
D. To expect more bad things
E. I just can't win

3. How has kidney disease changed you?

A. For the better
B. I gained some new strengths
C. It didn't change me
D. I'm worse off than before
E. It practically destroyed me

4. How often might things like this happen to you in the future?

A. Never
B. Hardly ever
C. Sometimes
D. Often
E. Constantly

5. How often do these things happen elsewhere in your life?

A. Never
B. Hardly ever
C. Sometimes
D. Often
E. Constantly

Are most of your answers A's and B's? If so, this is a good sign that you are learning from your kidney disease and making the best of it. Your positive attitude will serve you well. If you answered mostly C's, your attitude is neutral—not positive, but not negative either. You may be happier if you can seek out some meaning. If you had mostly D's and E's, you are having a rough time. It's as if you were singled out for bad things to happen to, and expect worse news in the future. Remember, you *do* have a choice about how to feel. If you can't find a positive way to look at what has happened and what you've learned, ask for help. Find someone to talk to who can help you see things in a different light. This is called "*reframing*" and it can make a huge difference in how you feel. How you talk to yourself can affect how you feel, too. A therapist can help you learn to change negative thoughts to more positive ones.

What hasn't seemed to be helpful to other people with kidney disease is to ask, "why me?" Why *not* you? The truth is that bad things happen to good people every day. **Kidney disease is not a punishment**. It's an illness with treatments that can help you have a full life, perhaps for decades. Looking back and saying, "I wish I'd appreciated what I had before" doesn't help you, either. But finding or setting up something to look forward to, and something else after that, can create a real improvement in how you feel about your life.

Setting Life Goals

Sometimes in the course of getting through one busy day after another, we can lose track of our dreams: what we want out of life. What we want to do for others. What we want to achieve or be or do. Here's your chance to take a few moments and think about your dreams. What inspires you in life? What gives you the most joy? What are you looking forward to?

Check as many as apply:

- ☐ Caring for my children or grandchildren
- ☐ Being there for a loved one who needs me
- ☐ Seeing my _____ get married
- ☐ Sharing a special birthday or event
- ☐ Watching a loved one graduate from high school or college
- ☐ Getting a high school diploma, or a college or graduate degree
- ☐ Helping people with _____
- ☐ Taking a trip to _____
- ☐ Getting a promotion at work
- ☐ Winning the lottery
- ☐ Holding a holiday celebration
- ☐ Being famous
- ☐ Going to a family reunion

Can you list at least one goal that you can work toward? If so, you have a focus for your life, and a reason to overcome this health setback and move forward. You can make your goal a reality by breaking it into small steps. Find someone to help you, and set a timeline for yourself. If you can't list at least one goal, you may be depressed and feel as if your life is over. That doesn't have to be the case. Read on.

Dealing with Depression

If you're feeling depressed about your illness, you have a lot of company. Depression is common in people who have *any* chronic disease, and even in healthy people. In a study of more than 5,000 people on dialysis in the U.S. and Europe, one in five said they felt down in the dumps or downhearted and blue.[1] Most of the day, we don't have strong emotions. Our mood is neutral; not good or bad, just *there*. With depression, your mood is down all the time, and you may struggle to get through a day. It is almost as if the air has turned into molasses. Depression can sap your strength and make you feel as if there is no light at the end of the tunnel. Feeling sad is not the same as being depressed. Depression symptoms last at least 2 weeks. Answer the questions on the next page if you think you might be depressed.

Are You Depressed?

These questions can help you find out. Please answer them by placing a "√" in the appropriate box.[2-6]

During the PAST WEEK, how often did you feel or behave this way?	Less than 1 day (rarely or none of the time)	1-2 days (some or a little of the time)	3-4 days (occasionally or a moderate amount of time)	5-7 days (most or all of the time)
I was bothered by things that usually don't bother me.	☐ 0	☐ 1	☐ 2	☐ 3
I had trouble keeping my mind on what I was doing.	☐ 0	☐ 1	☐ 2	☐ 3
I felt depressed.	☐ 0	☐ 1	☐ 2	☐ 3
I felt that everything I did was an effort.	☐ 0	☐ 1	☐ 2	☐ 3
I felt hopeful about the future.	☐ 3	☐ 2	☐ 1	☐ 0
I felt fearful.	☐ 0	☐ 1	☐ 2	☐ 3
My sleep was restless.	☐ 0	☐ 1	☐ 2	☐ 3
I was happy.	☐ 3	☐ 2	☐ 1	☐ 0
I felt lonely.	☐ 0	☐ 1	☐ 2	☐ 3
I could not get "going."	☐ 0	☐ 1	☐ 2	☐ 3

Score (Add up the tiny numbers below each box): ☐

What score did you get? A score higher than 14 means that you may have severe depression. It's wise to seek help if this is the case. You can feel better. Even a score in the 10-14 range means you may have some degree of depression. Please don't suffer if you don't have to. Talk to your social worker. He or she can counsel you or refer you to someone who can.

Feeling tired can make depression worse. Improving your energy level through exercise, better sleep, and treating symptoms like *anemia* (a shortage of red blood cells that can make you feel exhausted) can help a lot. It may sound backwards to say that you should exercise if you feel tired and depressed. But reams of studies prove that exercise can lift your mood and give you more energy. Don't think of your energy level as a flashlight battery that gets used up. Think of it as a *rechargeable* battery. Exercise is the power source that recharges your batteries. Talk with your doctor and start slow. See Chapter 14 for resources about how to exercise safely with kidney failure.

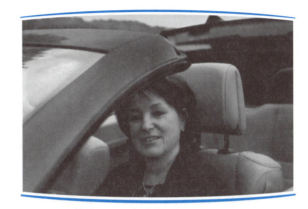

This is key: if you are depressed, choose a treatment that will *let you live more like you want to.* Putting yourself back in the driver's seat of your own life can make the biggest difference of all. It's not a surprise that you might feel depressed if your life has gotten away from you. *No one likes to feel powerless.* You are taking steps to help yourself by reading this book. Becoming your own expert will boost your coping skills and help you take back your life. You have options. Read on, and we'll tell you about them.

Fear of Death

In our work with people who have kidney failure, most thought they were going to die from it. One man who'd been on dialysis for *17 years* still felt as if at any moment he might just keel over. That was back in 1999. At the time of this writing in 2011, he's still here! In the 1990s, we did a research series of 90 phone interviews with people who had kidney failure. In these calls, some of the stories stood out, like:

- The man who never bought a home because he didn't think he'd live long enough to pay off a mortgage.
- The woman who was in college when she found out her kidneys were failing, and broke off her engagement—then had her tubes tied because she thought she could never have children.

Both of these people made choices without getting the facts first. Some women with kidney failure do have healthy babies. We know some who have. And there is no guarantee that *any* of us will live long enough to pay off a mortgage!

It's very normal to fear that life won't be worth living on dialysis, or that you'll die. But we found that most people never asked, they just *assumed* they knew what to expect. Sometimes they just "knew" based on loved ones on dialysis in the past. But times change. Medicine changes. And there are far better treatment options now for you than there were even a few short years ago.

How long might you live with kidney failure? That depends quite a bit on:

- **How old you are** – younger people tend to live longer on dialysis than older ones.

- **Your health history** – if kidney failure is your only health problem, you will likely live longer than if you have many other health issues, too.

- **How you take care of yourself** – this one is wholly under your control. If you choose a better treatment (some are better than others), stay positive, learn all you can, and follow your treatment plan, you will improve your chances of living longer—and better.

In a very real way, you are a survivor right now. The health problems that cause most kidney failure also tend to damage the heart. Most people succumb to heart problems before they can live long enough for their kidneys to fail. You are stronger than you know! When we cover each treatment in Chapters 6–9, we'll include what we know about life expectancy.

In another very real way, dialysis gives you the gift of being able to decide when to go. If you ever reach a point where your quality of life is no longer good, you can decide to let go by stopping your treatments. One 72 year old found this comforting:

"I can choose to die with dignity with compassionate support and palliative medical care. Why? Because my kidneys have failed. I am on dialysis. I can end my dialysis and check into a hospice whenever I choose, sooner or later slipping into the blissful fog that comes with death from kidney failure, though I am not planning on choosing to do so any time soon."[7]

If you ever reach a point where your quality of life is no longer good, you can decide to let go by stopping your treatment. This is not a choice most people have. If you have ever known a loved one who did not have a good death, you know what a gift this can be. Most faiths think of this as "letting nature take its course" by stopping life support—not as suicide. You can get "palliative care"—help for your symptoms, pain pills if you have pain—and you can choose what care you do or do not want. A hospice program can offer wonderful support and care for people whose doctors certify that they have 6 months or less to live.

It's best for *all* of us—with or without kidney failure—to write up an "advance directive." There are two types: a living will, and a durable power of attorney. Be sure that your loved ones know your wishes and have copies. This way, you can be sure that your wishes will prevail if you are too ill to speak for yourself. Most dialysis clinics want to know that people have advance directives.

What Kidneys Do for You

KEY POINT
Kidneys keep a constant internal environment in your body: *homeostasis*. Your treatment needs to mimic this balance for you to feel your best.

Good health is all about balance. This chapter contains details about how healthy kidneys work. You may want to read it word for word, skim it—or just read the key point and come back later.

All of the tissues and cells of your body are filled with and bathed by a kind of "primordial soup." Above all else, the role of the kidneys is to sense, monitor, and adjust this soup. Healthy kidneys keep the soup tightly controlled, and tweak the minerals, salts and fluids that make it up. If you get a soup recipe wrong, say, by adding too much salt, it tastes awful. In the body, if the make-up of the *intracellular* (inside the cells) and *extracellular* (outside the cells) soup is out of balance, no part of your body works as well. Keeping *homeostasis*—a constant internal climate in your body—is what healthy kidneys do.

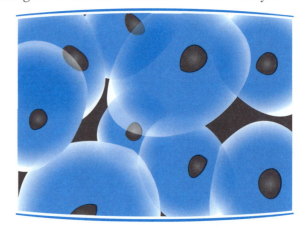

The more your treatment mimics homeostasis, the better you'll feel and the longer you may live. This is why a transplant is better at prolonging life than standard in-center dialysis.

Your Kidneys

Most people have two kidneys, each about the size of a closed fist. People may be born with no kidneys, just one, three or more, or two kidneys fused into a horseshoe shape. The kidneys are on either side of the back of the spine at about waist height. They have a tough outer capsule to protect a complex inner network of sensors, filters, and vessels.

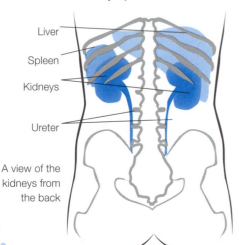

Liver

Spleen

Kidneys

Ureter

A view of the kidneys from the back

Each beat of your heart pumps blood through the main artery that runs through your belly—the *abdominal aorta*—and into your kidneys. Every five minutes, your whole blood volume passes through them. Sensors in healthy kidneys test each drop of blood for levels of water, minerals, salts and wastes. First, the kidneys remove wastes and excess water from the blood. Then, filtered fluid and wastes pass through tubes (*ureters*) and into the bladder as urine. Substances the body needs stay in the blood. This goes on 24 hours a day, 7 days a week.

Each kidney has from 300,000 to 1.5 million filters called 'nephrons'. Each nephron has two parts: a filter, called a *glomerulus* and a twisting, turning *tubule*. Tubules let substances out into your urine or reabsorb them so they stay in your body. The tubules empty into a tissue 'bag' on the side of the kidney called the renal pelvis. The renal pelvis leads, on each side to the ureters, and then to the bladder.

Homeostasis and Water Balance

So...why don't we swell up like water balloons if we gulp down a quart of lemonade on a hot day? Or shrivel up like raisins when we sweat hard? In healthy people, the brain and kidneys work together to keep you in homeostasis and ensure *euvolemia*: the same amount of water comes into the body and goes out.

This kidney brain team depends on a minute-to-minute sensing of the level of salt in your blood. This "sensing" is done in your brain. When blood salt levels rise or your blood pressure goes up, a hormone (*urodilatin*) tells your kidneys to let out more salt and water as urine.

Losing a lot of water through sweating or, say, a stomach flu, makes your blood more salty. This triggers your brain to release a hormone (*antidiuretic hormone*, or ADH). ADH tells the kidneys to hold onto water so you make less urine. And, it makes you thirsty so you drink more. Besides these hormones, each nephron has cells that check levels of salt and water in your blood.

In the body, all of these things go on each minute of each day. Each control must be in sync with all the others. Between them, a balance is kept: enough water and salt vs. too much or too little.

You can see what a complex system the kidneys and brain have worked out.

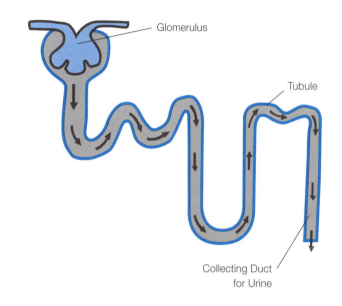

Glomerulus

Tubule

Collecting Duct for Urine

A Behind the Scenes Look at Blood Pressure Control

As part of salt and water balance, kidneys help control blood pressure. When blood pressure falls, less salt is sensed. This triggers a complex set of events:

1) *The kidneys release an enzyme (renin).*

2) *Renin tells the liver to release a peptide (angiotensin I).*

3) *A second enzyme in the lungs (angiotensin converting enzyme, or ACE), turns angiotensin I into an active form: angiontensin II.*

4) *Angiotensin II acts to shrink small arteries—which raises blood pressure.*

ACE inhibitor drugs lower blood pressure by blocking ACE, so no angiotensin II can form. A class of blood pressure drugs called angiotensin receptor blockers (ARBs) are close relatives of ACE-inhibitors and have much the same effect.

Fluid in Your Body

Each cell of your body is a tiny, living building block. Cells make up your tissues and organs. Think of a watermelon. It *looks* solid. If you dropped one on your foot, you would say it feels solid, too! Yet, a watermelon is 97% water.[1] Like a watermelon, cells have structure, but they are mainly water. The water that makes up the bulk of your body is **intracellular**—*inside* your cells.

Your cells live in a soup that keeps them fed and happy. This soup is **extracellular** fluid, the fluid *outside* your cells. (It is also called interstitial fluid.)

Your blood is a mix of water, salts, proteins, and cells:
- **Red blood cells carry oxygen**
- **White blood cells form part of your immune system**
- **Tiny platelet cells help your blood to clot if you have an injury**

Blood carries oxygen and nutrients to feed your cells. It also carries away wastes your cells make as they do their daily work.

Think of your body as a city. Your blood vessels are the roads: highways, lanes, and alleys, full of cars and trucks. Red blood cells bring goods and services. White blood cells are police and fire. And proteins and other carriers are the garbage men.

Single cells are the people in your city. They work alone and in groups. In a real city you might call these groups organizations. In the body, we call them organs.

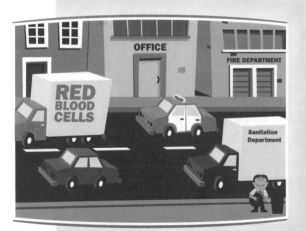

Your home, office, and suburb form your support systems. They are the **interstitium** that surrounds and nurtures you. It is the interface between you and the roads that bring your goods and take away wastes. Anything you need or want to throw out must use the road system. It must be brought into or out of the house or office. This can be a quick drop-off or pick-up, like an empty bottle to throw away. Or, it can be slow and difficult: a piano to get up to a top floor, or a king-sized bed to wrestle up the stairs.

It is the same in your body. Cells are fed and cleansed by substances that go back and forth through the interstitium. The interstitium is fed and cleaned by the bloodstream.

Any wastes your cells make must pass into the interstitium and then into the blood, so they can be carried away.

When the salt level of your blood changes, it triggers a cascade of water movement in your body. Water does not just slosh around inside you. It is held captive in three "spaces":

- **Intracellular space** – *inside cells (about 70% of body water)*
- **Interstitial space** – *between cells (about 20% of body water)*
- **Vascular space** – *in the bloodstream (about 10% of body water)*

Your body wants and seeks *equilibrium*: the *same* level of water and salt in all three spaces, all the time. This is a key point: Water shifts slowly from one space to the next to keep you in balance. Here's how it works:

1. The salt level in your blood goes up.
2. Water shifts from between your cells into your blood.
3. This shift of water goes on until your blood and your cells have equal salt levels.
4. Then, water shifts from inside your cells to the space between them, until salt is in balance there, too.

Restoring balance takes time. This process, called **osmosis**, goes on over and over in the course of a day. Keeping the right level and mix of salts in your blood at each moment is a key part of homeostasis. **Differences, called *gradients*, between levels of salt 1) in your blood, 2) between your cells, and 3) in your cells force water to shift until water levels in all three sites are the same. This shifting is called *osmosis*. In dialysis, water is removed from the blood using osmosis.**

Homeostasis and Electrolytes

Kidneys control minerals or salts in your blood called *electrolytes*. When dissolved, salts form *ions*: they carry an electrical charge. Your body is 50–60% water that is as full of salts as the sea. Your cells talk to each other through electrical signals carried by salts.

You take in salts (sodium, chloride, potassium, magnesium, calcium, and phosphate, to name a few) in foods you eat. You lose salts in body fluids like sweat, urine, vomit, diarrhea, and blood. Your body wants to always stay in balance, and kidneys make this happen.

We've listed the six main electrolytes healthy kidneys keep in balance. Testing labs may vary in how they measure these levels, so the values they quote as "normal" can differ a bit. This doesn't mean there is a real difference in the levels in the body. The levels we list in the chart as the high and low ends of the "normal range" for each one may not quite match up with the lab your blood tests go to. Don't panic if your levels are not exactly within normal limits. Talk with your dietitian, nurse, and doctor about how to bring them into the normal range for you.

Table 3-1: Electrolytes

Electrolyte	What it Does	"Normal"	Too Much	Too Little
Sodium (Na)	Controls how and where water goes in your body.	135 to 145 mEq/L	*Hypernatremia* – weakness, seizures, coma	*Hyponatremia* – brain swelling
Chloride (Cl)	Helps keep water levels in your body in balance.	96 to 106 mEq/L	*Hyperchloremia* – weakness, nausea, headache, sudden heart failure	*Hypochloremia* – Confusion, paralysis, or may have no symptoms
Potassium (K)	Vital for normal cell function. Helps send nerve signals and causes muscles to contract, including your heart.	3.5 to 5.3 mEq/L	*Hyperkalemia* – cardiac arrest, sudden death, or may have no symptoms	*Hypokalemia* – weakness, fatigue, muscle cramps, changes in heart rhythm
Magnesium (Mg)	Supports *enzymes*— proteins that speed up chemical reactions. Needed for all life.	1.4 to 2.1 mEq/L	*Hypermagnesemia* – trouble breathing, sleepiness, problems with heart rhythm, death	*Hypomagnesemia* – nausea, vomiting, weakness, painful foot cramps, tiny muscle twitches or tremors
Calcium (Ca)	Helps nerves signal muscles, helps activate enzymes, helps blood clot.	8.8 to 10.4 mEq/L	*Hypercalcemia* – thirst, fatigue, bone pain, stomach upset, confusion, seizures, changes in heart rhythm	*Hypocalcemia* – numbness of the fingertips and around the mouth, twitching, cramps, shortness of breath
Phosphate (PO$_4$)	Helps form cell membranes and aids energy transfer.	2.5 to 4.5 mEq/L	*Hyperphosphatemia* – phosphate can bind with calcium into sharp crystals that can form in soft tissues, causing pain, gangrene, or death	*Hypophosphatemia* – loss of appetite, muscle weakness, coma, and death

Healthy kidneys also control levels of bicarbonate (HCO_3). You might recall the pH test strips in school that turned pink or blue when you dipped them in an acid or a base. In healthy people, urine is a little acidic (pH of 6), and blood is a little basic (pH of 7.35 – 7.4). Bicarbonate is a buffer that helps keep the balance between acids and bases in the body and blood.

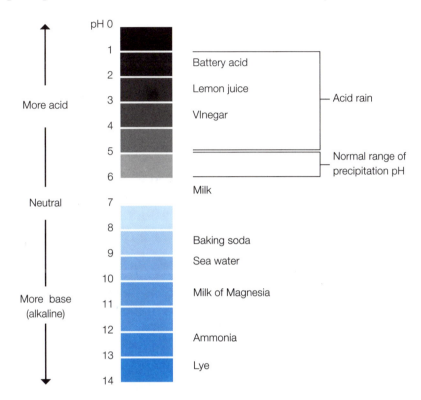

More acid

Neutral

More base (alkaline)

pH 0

Battery acid

Lemon juice

Vinegar

Acid rain

Normal range of precipitation pH

Milk

Baking soda

Sea water

Milk of Magnesia

Ammonia

Lye

Homeostasis and Wastes

Along with the liver and gut, the kidneys are your body's garbage trucks: they get rid of wastes. Wastes form when you eat or drink, break down drugs, or even move your muscles. It is easier to remove small wastes from the blood than large ones. Below, you can see why: large wastes aren't just big, they are also twisty and complex. It is harder for them to fit through pores (holes) in the cell walls to get out of the body.

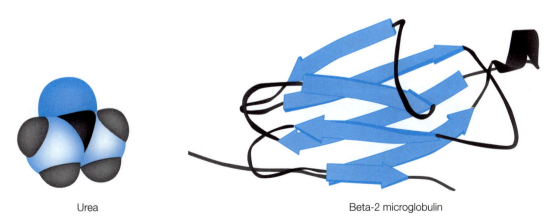

Urea

Beta-2 microglobulin

Small vs. Large Wastes

A 2005 study[2] found more than 90 wastes healthy kidneys remove. These wastes fell into four groups, based on molecular weight or size of the wastes, and whether the wastes were or were not bound to proteins:

Small molecules – There were 68 of these, including:

- **Urea**, a tiny protein waste that is very easy to remove. Urea is used to measure how "adequate" a dose of dialysis is (see "Adequacy: Don't be Fooled" in Chapter 6), though it does little harm by itself.
- **Creatinine**, a waste that forms each time you move your muscles.
- **Phosphate**, a unique small molecule, that acts like a middle molecule. It is twisty and hard to remove with dialysis. Since it is found in cells, between cells, and in the bones, levels rebound quickly, even during a dialysis treatment.
- Wastes with names like **putrescine** and **cadaverine** cause cell death (this includes red blood cells).

Middle molecules – There were 10 of these. The best known is beta-2 microglobulin (B2M), which causes a waxy protein called amyloid to form. Dialysis-related amyloidosis (DRA) can cause bone and joint problems after many years on dialysis. Other middle molecules include signal proteins (cytokines) like:

- **Interleukin-1**
- **Tumor necrosis factor**
- **Interleukin-6** – which can tell the body to make more B2M
- **Leptin**, a hormone that helps control body fat

Large molecules – There were 12 of these, but they were not listed in the article.

Protein-bound molecules – Some 25 of the solutes (28%) are bound to proteins. These solutes are small but hard for dialysis to remove, because the proteins to which they are attached tend to be large. Wastes found in the study include:

- **Indoxyl sulfate**, which causes scarring of the kidney filters.
- **Hippuric acid**, which makes drugs more toxic and increases insulin resistance.
- **Homocysteine**, which can damage the heart.
- **P-cresol**, which causes damage to the nerves, lungs, liver, and kidneys and can trigger seizures in people with epilepsy.
- **Advanced glycation end products (AGEs)**, which occur when sugars caramelize. They cause inflammation and can make heart and kidney disease worse.

When we talk about how dialysis works in Chapter 5, you'll want to think about how many of these wastes a treatment can remove. Wastes that stay in your body can poison your nerves, joints, and bones.

Homeostasis and Bone Balance

The kidneys help keep bones healthy. They work hand in hand with four small glands in the neck called the parathyroid glands. A complex feedback loop exists between the *parathyroid glands* in your neck and your gut, bones, and kidneys.

Parathyroid glands have one job: to keep your blood calcium levels in a tight range all the time. They sense calcium levels in your blood. If calcium is low, they churn out parathyroid hormone (PTH) and send it through your bloodstream. PTH does three main things.

1. **PTH tells your bones to let calcium out into your blood.** At a microscopic level, bones are remodelled all the time. Old bone is eaten away. As this occurs, calcium, phosphorus, and magnesium are set free from their bone storage and enter your blood. New bone is then made by bone forming cells.

2. **PTH sends the signal to convert vitamin D into its active, potent form.** Vitamin D you take in from foods (like dairy) is inactive. *Active* vitamin D lets your gut absorb calcium from foods. Without it, no matter how much calcium you eat, your body can't absorb or use it.

3. **PTH tells the kidneys to keep calcium in the blood and to excrete more phosphate.**

If this feedback loop is stopped, the result can be weak, frail bones that are easy to break.

Homeostasis and Oxygen Balance

It may seem odd to think that the kidneys affect how your body uses oxygen, but they do. Each cell in your body needs oxygen. Each time you breathe, you take in oxygen through your lungs, and it travels to your cells through nearly 100,000 miles of blood vessels, which include 40 billion tiny capillaries.

Doughnut-shaped red blood cells carry oxygen to each cell in your body. Ever wonder why they're red? They are filled with a red iron pigment called *hemoglobin*, which binds to oxygen. As red blood cells pass through the lungs, each one picks up oxygen. Then, when they squeeze one by one through your capillaries, they release their oxygen cargo to nearby cells. In this way, each cell in your body is fed oxygen.

Kidneys sense the level of red blood cells in the blood. If these levels are too low, the kidneys make a hormone called *erythropoietin* (EPO). EPO travels through the bloodstream to the bone marrow and tells the bone marrow to make more red blood cells. It takes a few weeks for red blood cells to grow large enough to do their job well.

The Balancing Act

All in all, you can see how vital the kidneys are for keeping your body in balance. We'll talk about how the loss of homeostasis and symptoms come together in Chapter 4.

When Kidneys Fail – Symptoms from the Loss of Homeostasis

KEY POINT

Restoring homeostasis with your treatment can help reduce symptoms so you will feel better and may live longer.

Your cells, tissues, and organs all talk to each other through your bloodstream. When kidneys keep your blood clean and your internal climate constant, this lets the rest of your body work as well as it can.

A treatment that is *physiologic* works the way your body does. Carl Kjellstrand, a nephrologist and PhD, wrote about the *unphysiology hypothesis* back in 1975.[1] He found that during dialysis, the wilder the swings in the water content and chemistry of the blood, the more symptoms people had. *The wilder the swings, the worse the symptoms.* The more normal blood volume and chemistry were, the better people felt. This should be no surprise. It is simple common sense!

The symptoms of kidney failure, called *uremia*, come mainly from the loss of homeostasis. How well you feel from one day to the next will depend on the kind and amount of treatment you get. If your treatment *brings back homeostasis*, most or all of your CKD symptoms will go away. Having fewer symptoms means you'll feel better from day to day and your long-term quality of life will improve. More physiologic treatment can also help you live longer.

Figure 1, shows you what *unphysiology* looks like using standard hemodialysis done for 3–4 hours three times a week. You can see the huge spikes in water and waste as they build up from one treatment to the next. The white shaded bar across the middle of the graph is the "average" range of homeostasis. This is

Figure 1

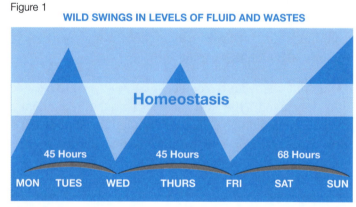

WILD SWINGS IN LEVELS OF FLUID AND WASTES

Homeostasis

45 Hours   45 Hours   68 Hours

MON   TUES   WED   THURS   FRI   SAT   SUN

where normal kidneys keep our internal "soup." You can see how far the levels of wastes and fluid go from normal as they build up between standard in-center HD treatments (in this case, on Monday, Wednesday, and Friday).

In contrast, Figure 2 shows what *physiologic* dialysis looks like – when dialysis is done nearly every day. You can see that the spikes in fluid and waste are now very small. In fact, most levels stay within the normal range all the time. No wonder people feel better!

To help you see what it means to have more vs. less physiologic treatment, here are some of the problems people with kidney failure complain about in the *short term*. We know this list is scary. You may not have all—or even ANY—of these symptoms! But we do want you to know what to watch out for and report to your care team. You'd be surprised at how many people don't know that the problem they're having is a "symptom" that can be helped. You might like to check off any that you feel you have had:

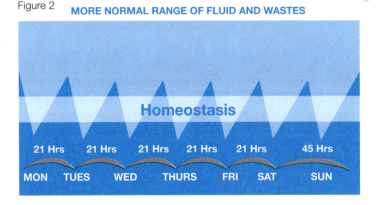

Figure 2   **MORE NORMAL RANGE OF FLUID AND WASTES**

Homeostasis

| 21 Hrs | 21 Hrs | 21 Hrs | 21 Hrs | 21 Hrs | 45 Hrs |
| MON | TUES | WED | THURS | FRI | SAT | SUN |

☐ **Swelling**. This is a symptom you notice if you have it. Water your kidneys can no longer remove builds up in your tissues. If you are on your feet a lot, you might have swollen calves, ankles, or feet that won't fit in your shoes. If your blood protein (*albumin*) levels are also low, your hands may swell and your rings may not fit. Your face may swell under your eyes.

☐ **Shortness of breath**. Water can build up in your lungs, too. Some people go to the emergency room thinking they have asthma or pneumonia or the flu, and find out that their kidneys have failed. Having too much water in your blood (your doctor may call this "fluid or volume overload") can overwork your heart. It can cause or worsen *congestive heart failure*—the heart becomes weak and flabby, and is just not up to the task of pumping so much blood.

☐ **High blood pressure**. A rise in blood pressure can be a cause—or a result—of kidney problems. Having too much salt and water (volume) in your blood as the kidneys fail tends to raise your blood pressure, even if it was always low or normal before.

☐ **Severe itching**. There are many reasons for itching (called *pruritus*) with kidney failure.[2] One cause can be wastes, called cytokines, that build up in the blood and trigger an immune response. An artificial kidney (dialyzer) made of a plastic called polymethylmethacrylate (PMMA) takes out more middle molecules than a standard one.* In one study, a PMMA kidney helped reduce severe itching in 30 people.[3] But, PMMA is costly and not used much in the U.S. Other causes of itching include nerves that are extra "jumpy," dry skin, and drug allergies.[4] The bone minerals calcium and phosphorus also get out of balance as the kidneys fail. Calcium phosphate crystals can form needle-like shards that lodge in the soft tissues and skin and cause itching. The higher the blood levels of calcium, phosphate, or worse, both, the more people itch.[5] The lower legs are most often affected. The itching can be very intense and may disturb sleep—and good sleep boosts survival.[6] *To learn more about middle molecules, read Chapter 3.

☐ **Loss of appetite**. You may have a bad taste in your mouth. A build up of wastes in your blood can make food taste like metal. And, you may find that you turn away from beef, chicken, fish, and other protein foods because they taste bad to you. The smell of food cooking may make you feel nauseous. Your breath may smell like ammonia. A loss of appetite can harm you: if you don't eat protein, you use up your body's protein stores, which can lead to malnutrition and muscle wasting. People who are malnourished on dialysis don't live as long.[7] The risk is even higher if you have other health problems besides kidney failure.[8] It is vital to eat enough protein, and good dialysis can give you the appetite to do that.[9]

☐ **Hair loss.** This problem is most often short term, but it can be very upsetting. Hair is made of protein, and it grows in cycles. After an active growth phase, hair follicles shrink and rest for 2–4 months. It is normal to lose 50–100 hairs per day. More loss than this is most often due to not eating enough protein. You may have been told to eat less protein while your kidneys were failing—or, you may have just not had any appetite for it. Most of the time, when you start dialysis and start to eat protein again, your hair will start to grow back after a couple of months. For people on hemodialysis, if hair loss persists, it may be due to a blood thinning drug called heparin.[10,11] Heparin is vital. It keeps blood from clotting in the artificial kidney (dialyzer) during a hemodialysis treatment. Changing to a different type of heparin or to a different blood thinner may help.

☐ **Fatigue.** A feeling of utter tiredness—fatigue—may come on as your kidneys fail. It can build slowly until it overwhelms you. One day, you may find that a walk across your home or up a short flight of stairs leaves you short of breath. While this can be due in part to a build-up of water or wastes, it is mostly caused by a shortage of red blood cells. Failing kidneys make less of the hormone *erythropoietin* (EPO). The worse the kidney failure, the less EPO the kidneys make, and the fewer red blood cells there are to carry oxygen. Your cells are starved for oxygen, which saps your energy and leaves your skin, gums, and fingernail beds looking pale. You may crave ice, clay, or laundry starch (a problem called pica). A shortage of red blood cells is called *anemia*. In CKD, anemia is most often due to a drop in EPO.[12]

☐ **Fuzzy thinking.** Without enough oxygen, your thinking may become fuzzy. It can be hard to focus. You may not recall things as well as you did, or may just not feel mentally as sharp.

☐ **Sexual problems.** What led to your kidney problems in the first place? If the cause was an illness that affects *just* the kidneys—like a form of nephritis or polycystic kidney disease (PKD)—chances are, it won't have much effect on your sex life. But if your kidney failure is due to diabetes or high blood pressure, these health problems can also cause sexual problems for men[13-15] and women.[16-19] Some drugs, like beta blockers and diuretics for high blood pressure, or some antidepressants can cause erectile dysfunction (ED).[20] ED can be the "canary in the mine," a warning that there are problems with blood flow and, sometimes, the heart.[21] Treatment of the problem with exercise and meds can help ED.[22] In a study of 792 men with diabetes, the better the blood sugar control, the less ED they had.[23] Though no one quite knows why, the loss of homeostasis with kidney failure can also wreak havoc with sex hormones.[24] Both men[25] and women[26] may lose interest in sex (decreased libido) and may be less able to reach orgasm. Age itself can cause a drop in sexual interest. Issues with body image or pain control (such as for the joint pain of arthritis) can affect sexual response. So, too, can just feeling tired and washed out. It may help you to know that much of this can be treated. Hormones like testosterone, drugs like Viagra®, Cialis®, or Levitra® for ED or, if the kidneys fail, better dialysis, or a kidney transplant, can all help.[27]

☐ **Depression**. Add severe fatigue to a fear that your life is careening out of control, and you have a common mix that can lead to depression. If your main response to things is "I'm too tired," or "What's the use?" you may be depressed. Or, if you are sad or blue most of the time, or it feels like you have to walk through water or syrup instead of air just to get through your day, again, you may be depressed. Feeling irritable can go hand in hand with depression. Irritation may come along first, and you may not see that it's *you*. It may just seem that all of those around you are very *annoying* all of a sudden. The standard response to depression in people who are on dialysis is to tell them that they can get help through counseling, exercise, and meds. These can help. But we think you can go beyond treatments—you can *improve your life with better dialysis*, taking back control by doing as much as you can for yourself.

In the longer term, the loss of homeostasis can lead to other problems. Some of the *longer term* symptoms are listed below. Check off any of these that you have had, too:

☐ **Sleep problems**. When homeostasis fails, sleep problems become rampant. You may feel sleepy all day—or not be able to fall asleep at night or sleep through the night.[28-30] One study linked sleep problems to high levels of phosphate in the blood.[31] If you have *sleep apnea* (a problem where you stop breathing many times each night—and may snore very loudly), you may have poor sleep quality, waking often each night and feeling sleepy all day. Sleep problems can reduce your quality of life.[32, 33] Restless legs syndrome (RLS) and periodic limb movements in sleep (PLMS) are common in people with CKD and in those on dialysis. No one is sure what causes the "creepy-crawly" feeling that makes you feel as if you *must* move your legs. RLS and PLMS occur in the general population, but are much more common in people with kidney failure.[34] They may be due to a build-up of wastes in the blood, since a kidney transplant[35] helps—though sleep quality in people who have had a transplant is still not as good as that of healthy people.[36] Not a whole lot is known, yet, about the *why* of sleep problems in CKD—we are only just starting to learn.

☐ **Skin changes**. Kidney failure can change the skin. During an HD treatment, the flow of fluid in the blood vessels to the skin, called *microcirculation*, changes.[37] Skin may darken or look yellow. Nails may become thin and break easily.[38] *Bullous* (blister) skin problems may occur. Or, blood thinning drugs, steroid drugs, or CKD itself can lead to purple spots with bleeding under the skin, and skin that is easy to tear and slow to heal. These symptoms may be due to a problem called *pseudoporphyria*,[39] which has been treated with the drug Mucomyst®.[40-42] Other very rare but severe skin problems can also occur in people on dialysis. One is *nephrogenic systemic fibrosis* (NSF), a syndrome that has been linked to use of gadolinum contrast dye for MRI tests.[43] NSF causes thick skin, stiff joints, lung fibrosis, and heart damage, and can be fatal.[44] For this reason, the risks of MRI contrast tests in people with CKD must be weighed against the benefits. In some cases, an ultrasound can be done. Or, perhaps a different contrast dye can be used. Kidney transplant[45] and the cancer drug Gleevec®[46] may help NSF. Extracorporeal photopheresis is a treatment that uses a drug that reacts to ultraviolet light to help clean the blood, and this helps NSF, too.[47] Another rare skin problem is *cholesterol crystal embolism syndrome* (CCE), which can cause skin ulcers, fatigue, and fever.[48] CCE can *cause* kidney failure, too, and one study found that it could lead to restless legs syndrome.[49]

Causes and Stages of Kidney Disease

Two thirds of all kidney failure in the U.S. is caused by Type II diabetes, high blood pressure, or, the "double whammy" of both at the same time. Other common causes of chronic kidney disease (CKD) include:

- **Type I diabetes**
- **Genetic cystic diseases** like polycystic kidney disease
- **Glomerular diseases** (nephritis) that affect the filter units of the kidneys, like IgA disease, membranous nephropathy or focal segmental glomerulosclerosis (FSGS)
- **Other diseases** that affect the whole body, like lupus
- **Blockages or a backup of urine in the ureters** that carry urine from the kidneys to the bladder (obstructive uropathy or reflux nephropathy)
- **Repeated urinary tract infections**
- **Over use of non-steroidal anti-inflammatory drugs** (NSAIDs) such as ibuprofen, indomethacin or naproxen, or the use of compound pain-killing pills
- **Blockage of the artery to the kidney, or renal artery stenosis (narrowing).** This problem can cause high blood pressure, and surgery or placement of a stent to hold the vessel open may help
- **Multiple kidney stones**

CKD is "staged" based on the *glomerular filtration rate* (GFR). Each of your 2 million or so nephrons has a *glomerulus*, a tiny capillary blood vessel, tangled in a ball, that filters the blood. The output of all of the glomeruli is the GFR. Most often, the GFR is not tested. It is estimated using a formula based on age, gender, race, and the blood level of *creatinine* (a waste removed by healthy kidneys). The result is the estimated GFR, or eGFR. A normal GFR is 90–120 mL/min (milliliters per minute):

- **Stage 1 CKD** – GFR is **normal** (90 mL/min or higher), but there is known kidney damage
- **Stage 2 CKD** – GFR is **60–89 mL/min**, and there is kidney damage
- **Stage 3 CKD** – GFR is **30–59 mL/min**
- **Stage 4 CKD** – GFR is **15–29 mL/min**
- **Stage 5 CKD** – GFR is **less than 15 mL/min**

Once the GFR falls to 6–9 mL/min (or higher if there are symptoms), kidney replacement treatment (dialysis or a transplant) is needed to live. You can get on the list for a deceased donor kidney or be tested for a living donor kidney when your eGFR is 20.

☐ **Fertility issues**. Hormone problems can cause heavy, irregular, or absent periods in women whose kidneys have failed. It may help to use less heparin during your period if yours are heavy. Talk to your care team. On standard in-center HD, the tissues of the uterus start to *atrophy* (waste away).[50] If you are a woman and want to have a baby, you may want to get more dialysis *now*, not later. It is possible to carry a healthy child to term while on dialysis—though the pregnancy is high risk, and extra care will be needed.[51, 52] In men, kidney failure can lead to a lower sperm count.[27] The chance of having a healthy child is better with a kidney transplant or with more dialysis. However, you still need to use birth control if you are fertile and don't want to have a baby right now. We will talk about this issue more in the chapters that cover each treatment option.

☐ **Neuropathy**. Nerve damage can occur if your dialysis fails to give you a GFR greater than 12 mL/min.[53] Since standard HD only gives 10–15% of normal kidney function,[54] nerve damage is common in those who use this option. The hands or feet may tingle, burn, or feel numb. It may feel like you are walking on marbles. Nerve damage may occur if the blood potassium is too high.[55, 56] It has also been linked with too-high blood levels of a middle molecule called tumor necrosis factor alpha (TNF-alpha).[57] Dialysis removes vitamin B_6 from your blood,[58] and taking B_6 has helped some people with nerve problems.[59, 60] Dialysis removes zinc, too, and zinc tablets can help—with the bonus of also helping the sense of taste.[61] ***(NOTE: Take only vitamins and supplements your doctor prescribes to prevent a harmful build-up in your blood.)*** A kidney transplant or better dialysis that gives you a higher GFR should help stave off this problem. If the nerve damage has been caused by diabetes, transplant and more dialysis may not be able to reverse the damage.

☐ **Joint pain**. Fibrils of a waxy protein called *amyloid* build up in the soft tissues, joints, and bones if your dialysis does not remove enough beta-2 microglobulin (B2M). Healthy people don't have amyloid fibrils. Enzymes called lysosomal proteases take their fibrils apart, so their B2M levels range from 0.9–1.5 mg/L.[62] People who do standard in-center HD don't have enough enzymes, and their B2M levels are 10–50 times higher.[63] Amyloid breaks down the bones which can lead to bone cysts, fractures, and damage to joints.[64] You may be told that you have "arthritis", which is, after all, inflammation in one or more joints. But this arthritis may be *caused* by amyloid, which can be prevented or removed with more dialysis. Amyloid fibrils are complex and pleated, and take time to remove. Long treatments, like long, slow, overnight dialysis, are the only way to remove enough B2M to prevent damage. Having a lower level of B2M is clearly linked with a longer life.[65]

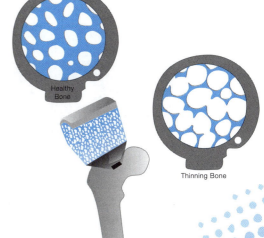

Healthy Bone

Thinning Bone

☐ **Bone disease**. As the kidneys fail, they become less able to keep bone minerals in balance. Bone disease has been found in nearly half of people with stage 3 or 4 CKD, and in nearly 2 out of 3 people with stage 5 CKD.[66] As we noted in Chapter 3, bones are remodelled all the time, driven in part by the kidneys. A tough outer coating of bone protects a lightweight honeycomb of thin inner bone, the bone marrow, and blood vessels. Too *much* remodelling can leave the outer layer too thin to do its job. Too little means new calcium isn't laid down to make the bones strong, so they are again too thin. Either way, bone pain, cysts, tumors, and fractures can occur. Bone can form *outside* the skeleton, too; a problem called *extraskeletal* *calcification.* This can lead to bony lumps in the brain,[67] eyes,[68] hands,[69] or any other part of the body. One man who had extra bone on his shoulder, hands, and feet had it melt away after 9 months of doing hemodialysis each night while he slept—because the longer treatments brought back the balance of bone minerals in his body.[70] Women can have osteoporosis and renal bone disease at the same time. In a randomized study, women on dialysis who were given the drug Miacalcin® (salmon calcitonin) had much better bone density at the spine and hip 3, 6, and 12 months later than the control group.[71]

- ☐ **Blood vessel calcification**. Heart disease and stroke are leading causes of death for most people in the U.S. That's also true for those with kidney failure.[72] When calcium and phosphorus are out of balance, bone can form in the blood vessels—even in the heart.[73] We don't know why, but smooth muscle cells in blood vessel walls *turn into bone-making cells* when the blood is not clean enough and calcium and phosphate levels have been too high.[74]

When calcium builds up, the walls of small and medium-sized arteries harden. Rigid blood vessels that can't stretch or shrink in response to changes in blood pressure raise the risk of a heart attack or stroke. Blood and oxygen flow to fingers and toes is poor, which creates a risk for gangrene and digit or limb loss.

Those who use standard in-center HD must take "phosphate binders" to help keep their blood phosphate from being too high. These meds lock up phosphate so it is removed in the stool and not absorbed. But, most binders are made with calcium—which can make the problems worse. And yet, studies with binders that *don't* have calcium have not shown longer life in those under age 65.[75]

What *has* helped? More dialysis.[76] Phosphate removal on frequent, nightly HD is so good that phosphate must be *added* to the dialysis fluid. In a study of people who did treatments every other night, 85.7% had less blood vessel calcification than they had on standard treatments.[77] Longer peritoneal dialysis treatments help, too.[78]

Calciphylaxis: Avoid a Lethal Problem

In a rare problem called *calciphylaxis*, crystals of bone block blood vessels and cut off the blood supply to tissues, limbs, and skin. Purple spots (most often on the legs) turn into skin ulcers that won't heal. The problem can lead to gangrene, loss of limb, or death. No one is quite sure what triggers the problem, though it is more common in people who have diabetes. The blood thinning drug warfarin has been linked with some cases that *look* like calciphylaxis, but are not.[79]

A drug called sodium thiosulfate—the antidote for cyanide poison—has been used to help calciphylaxis, alone or with other treatments.[80-82] (In rats, this drug keeps vessels from calcifying—but makes bones weak.[83])

Treatments that keep bone minerals in balance can help you avoid calciphylaxis and other forms of extraskeletal calcification. *Keeping your blood calcium level times your blood phosphorus level (called your "calcium-phosphorus product") at or below 55 can reduce your risk.[84]*

☐ **Left ventricular hypertrophy**. Your heart beats 70–80 times per minute pumping your blood through your blood vessels 24 hours a day, 42 million beats a year. Four chambers make this happen:

- Two *atria*, the right and the left, take blood into the heart from your veins.

- Two *ventricles* pump the blood out again through your arteries, on the right to your lungs, and on the left to the rest of your body.

Valves are "doors" that keep blood from backing up. They ensure a one-way flow. The "lub-dub" of a heartbeat occurs when your valves open and close. When the kidneys don't remove enough water from the blood, the muscle of the main pumping chamber can grow too thick. This is called *left ventricular hypertrophy*. LVH takes up space in the heart that is needed for the blood. This can lead to slow heart failure—or to sudden death.[85] As many as three out of four people on standard in-center HD have LVH[86,87]—a problem that starts early in kidney disease.[88] Diabetes adds to LVH; the left ventricle is not as strong, even when the degree of LVH is the same.[89] The main cause of LVH on dialysis *is too much fluid (salt and water) in the blood,* which raises the blood pressure.[90] Treatments that keep blood pressure low help prevent—or treat LVH.[91-96]

Did you check off any of these symptoms?

When we talked with people who have kidney disease, we found that many did not *know* they had symptoms until we gave them a checklist.[97, 98] In many cases, even if you have some of these problems now, it does *not* have to mean you will always have them. Bringing back homeostasis can send some of these problems packing!

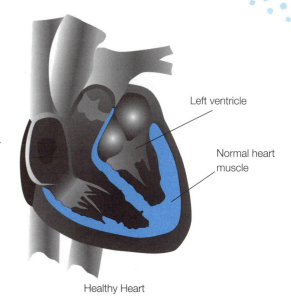

Left ventricle

Normal heart muscle

Healthy Heart

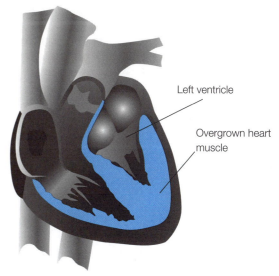

Left ventricle

Overgrown heart muscle

Heart with LVH

Any or all of these symptoms can be scary. But, what we aim to do in this book is show you how vital it is to get dialysis that brings you as close to homeostasis as you can get. When your body is in balance, you feel better. Your body works more like it should. And, if you get treatment that protects your bones, joints, and blood vessels, you'll need fewer drugs, spend less time in the hospital, and live longer, too.

So, when you choose a treatment, homeostasis is a key factor to keep in mind—no matter what other factors you need to weigh.

When to Start Dialysis

No-one wants the much-dreaded day to come, but one day it may. At least, after reading this book, you'll be ready. But, is it better to start dialysis early, while you still feel pretty well? Or to put it off as long as you can?

For a time, doctors believed it was better to start dialysis somewhat early—at an eGFR of, say, 10–15. But many of the more severe symptoms of uremia don't start until the eGFR drops to about 6. And, as it turns out, there is no benefit to starting early, IF you feel good and are not bothered by symptoms. There is a benefit to getting a dialysis *access* early—we'll talk about that in the next chapter. But waiting until you feel pretty bad won't shorten your life.

How do we know? In 2001, an article in the prestigious medical journal *Lancet* found that about 1 in 3 people chose to start dialysis late. After 3 years, the early starters did live about 2.5 months longer—but the late starters had an extra 4 months with no dialysis.[99] In 2002, the same authors reported that quality of life was higher for early starters in the first 6 months of treatment, but these differences disappeared after 12 months.[100]

Several more recent studies have found the same thing:

- The Australian Initiating Dialysis Early and Late (IDEAL) study was done from 2000–2008. Researchers randomly assigned 828 people to start treatment early vs. late. After 3–4 years, there were no significant differences between the groups in infections, complications, heart problems, or deaths.[101]

- A French study of 541 people done from 2005–2006 found that late starters had a higher risk of emergency dialysis starts and more illnesses. But they lived just as long as early starters.[102]

- A Swedish study observed 901 people who chose to start dialysis early or late. *Late starters were 84% more likely to survive than those who started early.*[103]

- A U.S. study found that an early dialysis start may be *harmful*. The researchers looked at survival in 81,176 people on standard in-center HD who did not have diabetes. *The risk of death went up the earlier dialysis began, from a low eGFR of 5.0–9.9 to a high of >15.* Those who started treatment with eGFRs of 5–9.9 were more than twice as likely to survive.[104]

Talk with your doctor. See what will be the best course of action for *you*.

How Dialysis Works

KEY POINT

Dialysis of any type needs a filter, a fluid called *dialysate*, and a special "access" to reach the blood.

If you've read Chapter 3, you know how healthy kidneys keep your body in balance. And if you've read Chapter 4, you know the sorts of symptoms that can occur when this balance is lost.

Dialysis is a treatment that filters wastes and excess water out of the blood of people whose kidneys have failed. The process requires a membrane, dialysate fluid, and a way to access the blood.

This is the longest chapter in the book. It covers a lot of ground, but when you're done, you'll know a LOT more about dialysis.

First, You Need a Membrane

Kidneys have built-in filters: nephrons. When they fail, you will need a new filter. The key part of this new filter is the *membrane*—a thin layer of tissue that forms a barrier.

Dialysis needs to *keep in* substances you need, like protein and red blood cells. And, it needs to *let out* ones you don't, like excess **water** and **wastes**. So, the membrane has to be *semi-permeable*—it needs to ensure that only wastes are removed. Permeability—*pore size*—of the membrane is key: some wastes are larger than others. A *high flux* membrane has bigger pores and can remove more "middle molecules" than a standard, low flux membrane.

How well a membrane will work depends on:

- What it is made of
- What its surface area (in meters^2) would be if it were laid out flat
- What size the pores are to let wastes through

Dialysis membranes are also used to remove excess water from the blood during dialysis. This is called *ultrafiltration*. Pressure from a pump is used to squeeze water out of the blood through the membrane.

It is best if the membrane is *biocompatible*: so much like your body that it does not cause an immune response. When your immune system meets a foreign body, it causes inflammation. White blood cells and other immune factors rush to your aid. When each treatment triggers this, it stresses your system. Inflammation:

- **Triggers blood vessel calcification** by blocking a protein (fetuin-A) that stops this problem in healthy people.[1]
- **Slows the rate of bone repair.**[2]
- **Requires higher doses of EPO to treat anemia**.[3]
- **Is linked with heart disease and malnutrition**.[4]
- **Changes microcirculation in the skin during treatment**, which can lead to skin problems.[5]

A blood test for C-reactive protein (CRP) is used to show if inflammation is present.

Which membranes are biocompatible?

Peritoneal dialysis (PD) uses the blood vessels and the single layer of cells called the *peritoneum* that line the inside of your abdomen as the membrane. Since these are part of your body, they are 100% biocompatible. (Read about PD in Chapter 7.)

In hemodialysis (HD), the membrane is a bundle of thousands of hair-thin hollow tubes inside a clear plastic tube. The membrane and tube are called a *dialyzer*, or artificial kidney. (Read about types of HD in Chapters 6, 8, and 9.) HD membranes are made of:

- **Cellulose acetate, diacetate, or triacetate** – these forms of cellulose from plants, like cotton, are changed to make them less likely to cause immune reactions. They are a bit higher flux and more biocompatible than plain cellulose, which is no longer on the market.
- **Polysulfone** – a costly plastic first used in 1965. Membranes made of polysulfone can be low or high flux, based on pore size.
- **Polyethersulfone** – a high flux, somewhat biocompatible membrane patented in 1990. Since it is lower cost, it is used in single use dialyzers.
- **Polyester polymer alloy (PEPA)** – a high flux membrane that is quite biocompatible. PEPA is used alone or with other plastics, and the pore sizes vary.
- **Polymethylmethacrylate (PMMA)** – you may have run across this by one of its common names: Plexiglass or Lucite. As a dialyzer membrane, PMMA is biocompatible and very high flux. In fact, it will even let wastes that are bound to proteins pass through. It is not yet in use in the U.S.

Coating a membrane with vitamin E can reduce the risk of inflammation.[6] So does reusing the dialyzer, since a coating of your own blood protein forms inside the membrane.[7] If reuse is done, the dialyzer must be sterilized before it is used again. Sterilizing with steam works better than using a chemical (ethylene oxide).[8] On the other hand, one study found bacterial DNA in a reused membrane.[9] This residue can cause a low level infection—with inflammation. There is good and bad in reuse, and debate about the risks and benefits of reuse goes on to this day.

Dialyzer reuse is common in the U.S. The main reason for reuse is cost control. Reuse also sends less waste to landfills. Reuse of dialyzers is no longer done in many other countries. Australia, where it is now against the law to re-use medical equipment (like a dialyzer), stopped doing reuse back in 1992. This is also true of many other western countries.

Blood is taken to and then back from the dialyzer through plastic tubing (often called *lines* by dialysis nurses). Blood can quickly clot when it is outside the body or touches plastic. *Heparin*, a blood thinning drug, is given during an HD treatment to help keep clots from forming in the dialyzer or tubing.

A Place for Wastes: Dialysate

In your body, your kidneys sorted out wastes and excess water and sent them to your bladder as urine. When you don't make much (or any) urine, you need a place for wastes to go. In dialysis, wastes and water pass out of the blood, across the dialyzer membrane, and into a fluid called *dialysate*, or "bath." Dialysate is a mix of water and chemicals.

Dialysate in Peritoneal Dialysis (PD)

For PD, dialysate comes in sterile bags. In most cases glucose (sugar) is used to pull wastes out of your blood. Three "strengths" of bags are made, based on the level of glucose, which is used to create a *gradient* (difference) between the fluid and your blood, to remove wastes:

- **1.5% glucose**
- **2.5% glucose**
- **4.25% glucose**

The higher numbers mean a stronger gradient—which is *much* harder on your body. Glucose is heated when PD fluid is made, and some of it turns into caramel, or "glucose degradation products" (GDPs). GDPs cause "advanced glycation end products" (AGEs) to form.[10] Over time, AGEs cause fibrosis of the peritoneal membrane, so it may no longer work for PD.[11] Use of stronger PD fluids with more glucose speeds up this process. In rats, a new drug called *alagebrium* helps break down AGEs.[12] Some day this drug or one like it may help in people, too.

Dialysate in Hemodialysis (HD)

Most of the "guts" of a dialysis machine aim at making sure the dialysate is clean, correctly mixed, heated to the right temperature, and free of air or impurities. You have learned that HD membranes have pores to let wastes out of your blood. This means there is also a chance that they can let *pathogens* (harmful bacteria, viruses, or fungi) *into* your blood, through *backfiltration*. So, it's not just the membrane that matters to your health—you also need clean water in your dialysate.

Tap water is safe to drink, because it is treated to kill most pathogens. Your stomach acid kills the rest. Water that *touches your blood* in the form of dialysate needs much more treatment. Water treatment for HD removes most pathogens, chlorine, heavy metals (like lead), and other things that could harm you, like:

- **Nitrates** – part of some fertilizers, these can keep your body from using oxygen.
- **Calcium & magnesium** – these minerals can cause "hard water syndrome"—nausea, vomiting, headaches, skin flushing, weak muscles, and blood pressure changes.
- **Sodium & potassium** – these are part of dialysate, and must be kept in precise amounts. Extra levels in water must be removed.
- **Sulfates** – this class of minerals can cause nausea and vomiting in people on HD.
- **Copper & zinc** – soft water can leach these toxic metals out of plumbing pipes or water cisterns. In the body, they can cause nausea and vomiting, liver damage, death of red blood cells, and other problems.
- **Heavy metals** – arsenic, barium, cadmium, chromium, lead, mercury, and selenium are poisons that can build up in the body.
- **Chloramines** – mixing chlorine and ammonia makes a toxic gas that is used to kill germs in drinking water. Chloramines are toxic for humans.
- **Aluminum** – can occur in nature or be added to make city water more clear. It can build up in the bones and brains of people on HD.
- **Fluoride** – added to city water to help prevent tooth decay, but harmful on HD.
- **Bacteria** – one-celled microbes that can cause disease. Bacteria form *biofilm* (slime) that lets them cling to wet surfaces.

How clean is clean?

If you do HD, your blood comes into contact with water in the dialysate. The cleaner the water is, the less it will trigger an immune response in your body. The U.S. has lower standards for dialysis water than other parts of the world—but some dialysis companies choose to exceed the U.S. standards.

- In the U.S., dialysate water can have up to 50 colony-forming units (CFU) of bacteria (live germs) in each milliliter (mL)—about 1/5 of a teaspoon.[13]
- There are 1,000 mL in a liter.
- A standard HD treatment may use 120 liters.
- Each treatment can put your blood in contact with 6 million bacteria.

Live bacteria are not the only risk. When bacteria die, toxic parts of their cell walls, called *endotoxin* break free. Endotoxin can cause fever and chills—a *pyrogenic* (fever causing) reaction. Smaller amounts of endotoxin can cause chronic inflammation.

U.S. dialysate can have 1.0 endotoxin unit (EU) per mL.[13] In one treatment, 120,000 bits of endotoxin may touch your blood. So-called "*ultrapure*" water for dialysis must reach a far higher standard. Each mL of ultrapure water must have less than 0.1 EU.[13] Using ultrapure water for dialysate has been shown to reduce whole body inflammation.[14] People who used ultrapure water had less B2M in their blood.[15] They needed less iron and EPO to treat anemia.[16] They had healthier hearts, too.[17]

Osmosis and Diffusion

Once you have a filter and dialysate, two principles make dialysis work. We talked about the first one, **osmosis**, in Chapter 3. In your body, water shifts from in your cells, to between your cells, and then into your bloodstream. This goes on until the water level in all three fluid spaces is equal.

We use osmosis in dialysis by adding salt or sugar to dialysate. This forms a *gradient* (difference) between blood on one side of the membrane and dialysate on the other. Water will shift out of your blood, through the membrane, and into the dialysate until both sides are equal. The used dialysate is then flushed down a drain.

Diffusion is similar—but removes wastes instead of water. Like water, *solutes* (dissolved wastes in your blood—like phosphate) shift from one fluid space to another until the levels are equal. Think of a tea bag. The tea leaves stay inside the bag, but the tea *diffuses* out into hot water. Dialysate has none (or very little) of the wastes you want to remove. The gradient causes wastes to move across the membrane into the dialysate. How much of each waste will come out depends on:

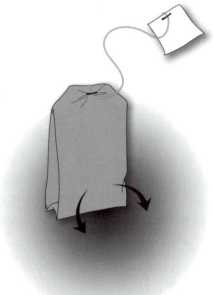

- The size of the molecule
- Pore size of the membrane
- How long a treatment lasts – small molecules are easy to remove; larger ones take longer
- What is in the dialysate
- How fast blood flows to the dialyzer

Blood Access

Dialysis, then, is a treatment that removes wastes and water from the blood, using diffusion and osmosis. How do you get to the blood? You need an "access." No matter what type of treatment you choose for kidney failure, some type of minor surgery will be needed to make an access.

If the thought of surgery scares you, it may help you to know that fear of needles and surgery is very common. Each year, people who share these fears get kidney failure and start dialysis. They have been able to overcome their fears. Your care team is there to help you. You CAN do this, and you will never be alone as you journey through dialysis. You can make choices about things like local vs. general anesthesia, or inpatient vs. outpatient that may help ease your mind. Talking to others who have been through the procedure you will need may also help. Read about needle fear on page 46, too, for some more ideas.

PD Access: Catheter

For peritoneal dialysis (PD), the access is a *catheter* (plastic tube). A surgeon places the tube through the wall of the belly or chest. The tube reaches into the peritoneum, the blood-vessel-rich lining of the inside of the abdomen. The peritoneum forms a sac, which is filled up with dialysate—using the tube.

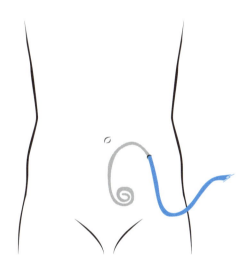

Your skin

Catheter tip

Abdominal PD Catheter Types

PD catheters are soft and flexible, and about the size of a drinking straw. They are made of polyurethane plastic or silicone rubber, with one or two Dacron® cuffs. One cuff is placed into your muscle wall. A second one may be placed in the skin at your *exit* site (where the catheter comes out of your body). Your own tissue will grow into the cuff(s) and help anchor the catheter in place. The cuffs also help keep germs from travelling up the catheter and into your body.

The tip of the catheter that is inside your body may be straight. Or, it may be coiled in a spiral, grooved, or have flat silicone discs to help hold your tissue layers apart to improve drainage. Many designs have been tried, and they all seem to have about the same results.[18] Ask your surgeon to show you the type you will have.

PD catheter placement in the abdomen is most common. The exit site is about an inch under the belly button. The catheter can be below your belly button or to the right or left of it. ***Tell your doctor where your belt falls so the catheter can be placed where it will not rub.*** The exit site should face down, so there is no "pucker" above the catheter where water and germs could collect. You must keep the catheter clean and dry to avoid infection. You can take a shower with an abdominal PD catheter, but not a bath. Most programs do not suggest swimming, though private pools may be okay.

Catheter placement is a quick (15–30 minute), minor procedure. It should be done in an operating room to help prevent infection. If you are nervous, ask about drugs to help you relax or sleep. You won't be able to eat after midnight, so you may want to set up your visit for the morning. The nurse or doctor will draw on your skin with a marker to show where the catheter will go. Some clinics will require you to have an enema and/or take a shower before the placement. You may be asked to use a special cleanser, like chlorhexidine, to remove germs from your skin. Just before the procedure, you will need to empty your bladder.

Abdominal PD Catheter Location

There are four ways to place an abdominal PD catheter:[18]

- **Surgical** – This is the most often-used (but most costly) approach. You will be given *local* (just the area) or light general anesthesia. A surgeon will make a tiny (1–2 cm) cut through your belly and the wall of the *peritoneum*, which lines your abdomen. S/he may pull out and remove some *omentum*, a curtain of tissue in the abdomen, so it does not get in the way of the catheter. Then s/he will push the catheter through the cut and stitch around it. The surgeon will choose an exit site and use a tunneling tool to make a place for the catheter under your skin. S/he will pull the catheter through the tunnel until the cuff is in the right place, then stitch around it.

- **Trocar** – Using local anesthesia, a surgeon will make a small (2–3 cm) cut through skin and muscle. PD fluid will be placed in your abdomen using a needle or tube. Then, you will be asked to tense your stomach muscles so a trocar (pointed tool) can be inserted. S/he will pull the *trocar* out and use the hole to place the catheter and stitch it in place. Then s/he will make a tunnel under the skin to an exit site, and stitch around it. Since a trocar makes a large hole, this technique may cause more leaking.

- **Guide Wire** – Using local anesthesia, a surgeon will make a small (1–2 cm) cut through skin and muscle. S/he will ask you to tense your stomach muscles so a small tube can be pushed through your peritoneum. PD fluid will be placed in your abdomen. The surgeon will put a guide wire through the tube, and use the wire to put the catheter in the right spot. Then the surgeon will make a tunnel under your skin to an exit site and place stitches around it. This technique may cause less leaking. But, there is a risk that the small tube could puncture your bowel.

- **Scope** – Using local anesthesia, a surgeon will make a small cut through skin and muscle. S/he will insert a mini-trocar with a thin tube inside through the wall of your abdomen. Then s/he will remove the trocar and insert a scope so s/he can see the inside of your abdomen. After the catheter is placed and stitched, the guide will be removed. The surgeon will make a tunnel under the skin to an exit site, and place stitches around it. A surgeon needs special training to use the scope.

Some surgeons will keep the catheter under the skin for two weeks or more, and not make an exit site. When it is time to start PD, the surgeon will make a small cut and pull the catheter out. This is called the *Moncrief-Popovich procedure*. Research suggests that this may help catheters last longer and lower the risk of infection.[19]

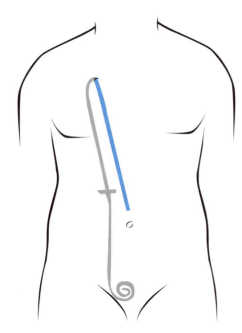

Presternal PD Catheter

A ***presternal catheter***[20] is placed into the chest wall, and the tip reaches down into the abdomen. The chest skin is thinner and less germy than the abdomen, so infection is less likely. Chest skin also moves less than belly skin, so a presternal catheter is a good choice for an active child or someone who is heavy. You can take tub baths with a presternal catheter, if you keep it out of the bath water. (Swimming is not suggested.) Presternal catheters are not offered all over the U.S. You may or may not be able to find them where you live.

Before you get a presternal catheter, you'll be asked if you prefer it to exit on the right or left side. If you are a woman, *avoid your bra area so the catheter will not rub*. You will be given antibiotics through an intravenous line within 24 hours of the time the catheter is placed. Using anesthesia, small (3–4 cm) cuts are made at the second and third rib and on the abdomen. Two parts of the catheter are inserted and held in place with a titanium connector. Pockets are made under the skin for the cuffs.

Ask for a Transfer Set

A "transfer set" is a 4–6 inch length of tubing with a titanium valve to let a PD catheter open and close. **Ask the surgeon to put on a transfer set in the operating room—it takes only seconds**. If this is not done, it may take 30–45 minutes to put one on in the dialysis clinic, and the risk of infection is quite a bit higher.

When you do PD, your transfer set will need to be changed every 6 months. This is a sterile procedure. It can be done in the dialysis clinic, or you can learn to do it at home.

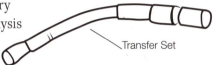

Transfer Set

How You May Feel Afterward

Most people tell us they don't feel much pain after having a PD catheter placed. Some are hungry because they had to fast for a few hours. Some get right up and walk and do not need any painkillers. Others do have some pain for 3–5 days, take pain pills, and find it hard to wear pants.

If you had general anesthesia, you may feel groggy afterward, and may have some nausea. Since you don't know how you will feel, it's wise to plan to take it easy for a few days so you can heal.

Caring for Your New PD Catheter

When PD fluid is placed in your belly during catheter placement, some may leak out and soak the bandages. You should be given clean, dry gauze and tape to take home in case this happens. Your belly may also feel tight if fluid was left in. This will ease up over time.

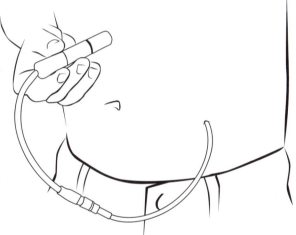

In most cases, your PD training nurse will want to change your dressings. This is a chance to check on how well your catheter is healing. Once your exit site looks good, you may be asked to leave off the dressings so it can finish healing in the open air.

At a clinic visit, your PD nurse will flush out your catheter with PD fluid to see how well it drains. To do this, the nurse will add a *tubing extension* onto your transfer set. Ask if you have a choice about length—it is easier to care for a shorter catheter. A bag of fluid will hang from an IV pole and drain into your belly through the catheter. Unless the fluid is cold, you may not feel this at all. If the flush goes well, you'll be ready for training. Often, training can start within a week or two after getting your catheter.

What Can Go Wrong?

No treatment is perfect. Any type of access—for PD or for HD—has its challenges. So, when you read this section, keep in mind that most of these issues can be prevented with good, careful technique.

One key to successful, long-term PD is keeping germs out of your catheter and your peritoneum. It isn't easy, because germs are all over. But in your training, you'll learn steps for *aseptic* (germ-free) technique that you'll need to follow closely. It will seem like a lot to learn at first, but the steps will quickly become a habit—like brushing your teeth—that you can do without thinking too much about it.

You can prevent nearly all PD catheter infections with careful attention to hygiene. Some types of infection that can occur with a PD catheter include:

- **Exit site infection** – This occurs when germs grow in the skin where your catheter comes out of your body. Some programs will have you use an antibiotic cream to prevent this. Mupirocin has been proven to reduce infection by about two-thirds.[21] Other programs will have you air-dry your exit site so it is not moist, since germs love warm, moist places. If you get an exit site infection, your doctor will prescribe antibiotics. An exit site infection can lead to a tunnel infection.

- **Tunnel infection** – If germs get into the tunnel under your skin where the catheter goes, the infection can be hard to get rid of—and it can reach the peritoneum. Your doctor will prescribe antibiotics, and you may need to get a new catheter if the infection does not clear.

- **Peritonitis** – Infection of the peritoneum can be very painful and can cause fever and internal scarring. In some cases, scarring can stop you from doing PD. You'll learn to watch for cloudy fluid and report pain right away so you can start antibiotics. (If you can't read newspaper print through used PD fluid, it is cloudy.) Some peritonitis is caused by fungal infections.

Sometimes PD catheters can leak. Fluid can leak out around the catheter and into the abdominal wall, draining down to swell the penis or scrotum in men or the labia in women. Sometimes this can be solved with a brief rest from PD. Other times, surgery is needed to fix the leak.

HD Access: Background

Hemodialysis (HD) needs a *vascular access*—a way to reach your blood vessels. To do a treatment, tubes take your blood to and from the dialyzer (more about this later). Today, there are three ways to access the blood for HD:

- **Fistula** – by far the best choice if you can have one
- **Graft** – a second best choice
- **Catheter** – this is not the same as a PD catheter—and not as safe for you

Doing HD with a fistula or a graft requires two needles. Catheters do not use needles—but they have other, severe problems. Solving the problem of how to reach the blood vessels for HD is what first made chronic dialysis possible. Veins are close to the skin's surface and easy to reach—but don't have enough blood flow for HD. Arteries are large and have a strong blood flow—but are too deep to reach. In the early days of HD, the doctor had to cut through the skin to reach an artery for each treatment. Once used, the artery had to be tied off and could not be used again. This meant that only about ten HD treatments could be done, so HD was for short-term use only. *Even now, there are only about ten sites on the body where an HD access can be made, so it's still vital to protect each one.*

So, what changed this? In 1960, Dr. Belding Scribner invented a U-shaped Teflon® shunt to link an artery and vein in the wrist. The shunt was wrapped with a bandage between treatments. It could last from a few days to a few years, and then be replaced. But, since the shunt was outside the body, it was quite prone to infection and clotting.

Scribner shunt

In 1966, Dr. James Cimino replaced the shunt with the first surgery to link an artery and vein *under* the skin. After a few weeks to mature, strong blood flow from the artery would "arterialize" the vein, making it large and strong enough to be used for HD. **Today, this arteriovenous fistula (AVF) is still by far the best type of HD access.**

HD Access: Fistula

Since a fistula is under the skin, it is less prone to infection. It resists blood clots, since it uses only your own blood vessels, which are lined with a smooth layer called *intima*. And, artery walls have muscles that snap shut after the HD needles are removed. This means fistulas *self-heal*, so they last longer. A healthy fistula will have a strong blood flow, and can last for decades. We know people who have used the same fistula for more than 30 years. People who use fistulas for HD tend to have healthier hearts and live longer than those who don't.[22]

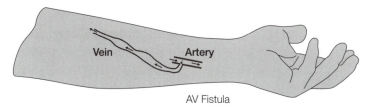

AV Fistula

Most—but not all—people can have a fistula. If you have a blood vessel disease, a pacemaker, or other health problems, a fistula may not work for you. **Ask for ultrasound vessel mapping to find out**—the surgeon can see your blood vessels through your skin with this painless test! One study found that three out of four people who had "poor veins" by exam alone were able to have a fistula when vessel mapping was used.[23] Medicare pays for vessel mapping, and other health plans may, too. Call your plan's customer service number to find out.

Get an Early Start on a Fistula

If you plan to do HD, it is best to get a fistula well before you need to start treatment—when your eGFR has dropped to around 20 mL/min (or about one fifth of normal). It is okay if a fistula works for a year or more before you need HD. Some people have a surgical problem getting a fistula up and running. Getting an early start buys you time to be sure your fistula works when you need it.

It may take more than one try to get *any* type of working access. For example, a fistula can be formed at the wrist, but your veins may be too small to allow it to mature enough to be used. If so, a second try may be at your elbow or upper arm. If your upper arm has a thick layer of fat tissue, your vein may be very deep. The vein can be *transposed*—moved closer to the surface of your skin. In Australia, this is called "superficialized" and about 1 in 3 fistulas is made this way. If any of this is the case for you, please be patient. A good, working fistula is key to your future life and health.

Choose a vascular (blood vessel) surgeon who has made as many working fistulas as possible. Ask your nephrologist to refer you, and know that the best surgeon may not be in your local area. Each doctor's success rate can vary, and you want the best. An access is your HD lifeline, and there is no substitute for a good lifeline. A recent study found that surgeons who did at least 25 fistulas while they were in training are best at making them work.[24] So, ask your surgeon how many fistulas he or she made as a trainee and about his or her success rate now. It may be worth a bit of travel to get a good lifeline.

What to Expect

You may have local or general anesthesia for fistula surgery—and you may get to choose which you would prefer. After surgery, you will need someone to drive you home. Your arm will be swollen, and you'll need to take pain pills for a few days. It takes at least 1 month and, ideally, 3–4 months for a fistula to *mature* enough to use for HD. This means the vein will grow bigger and the vessel walls will thicken. You can expect that:

- **Your fistula will vibrate, and you can feel a buzz**—this is called a *thrill*. You will learn how to feel each day for this healthy sign. A fistula with no thrill is a fistula in trouble. *Tell your care team right away. Don't wait.* Call the emergency number you were given if your clinic is closed.

- **Your fistula will have continuous whoosh-whoosh sound you can hear through a stethoscope** (called a *bruit*). If you have a stethoscope (you can buy one for $10 or so at a drugstore), you can listen to it. *If the sound gets higher in pitch—like a tea kettle ready to boil—or it stops, call the clinic or emergency number right away.*

- **Watch for any redness, swelling, drainage, or change in your fistula after it heals, and call your care team**.

- **Don't squeeze your fistula arm** with elastic, a tight watch, or by carrying something across it. You don't want to compress the fistula, it could cause damage to the vessel lining and cause narrowing.

- **Your doctor may suggest exercises**, like squeezing a rubber ball or a rolled up washcloth, to help your fistula mature faster.

- **You may need ultrasound exams** so any "mischief" can be detected early, such as a narrowing in the vein or a poor blood flow. If found, steps must be taken right away to fix the problem (perhaps with surgery). It is much harder to fix a non-working fistula than to step in and help one that has a problem but is still working. An X-ray dye test (*venogram*) may be used to pinpoint the trouble spot.

- **Some fistulas don't work.** It may take more than one try to get a working fistula. Don't give up!

A fistula (or a graft) can "steal" too much blood from the rest of your hand or arm. This problem is even called "steal syndrome." If you have steal syndrome, your hand might feel cool to the touch, turn white or blue, or ache when your access is used. In the short term, a warm glove may help ease the pain. But *talk to your surgeon*: you may need other vessels to be tied off or a revision of your access. You don't want to risk not getting enough blood to your hand. In very rare cases, people have lost a finger, hand, or arm due to a dialysis access problem that wasn't taken care of right away.

Your fistula will grow. If it works, a fistula will get bigger. So, the vein enlarging is a sign that your fistula is working. But, it can be hard to get used to. Besides a scar on your arm, you will have a large vein (it may grow up to about half an inch wide over time) that people can see. This is *normal* and it is the sign of a good, healthy lifeline. It can also be hard to come to terms with, especially if you did not expect it. In most ways, people who don't know you won't know that you are on dialysis, but a fistula can show.

Some people wear long sleeves year round to hide their fistula or graft. Others choose to look at their access as the battle scar of a war they are winning with kidney failure. After all, we *all* have our scars. Some use questions about their access as a chance to teach people something they didn't know about kidney failure. Or, they may make up a silly story ("a shark bit me") to silence those they don't want to talk to. If you expect this and know that it's normal, it may help you to cope with the change in your body when it occurs.

Dialysis Needles

"I had 3 fistula surgeries before we finally got one that worked. Once it matured, the nurses had trouble cannulating it and infiltrated me 3 times in a row. I kept asking how could they NOT feel it when I could feel it so well? Then, the next treatment, I asked if I could do it, no training, nothing. I just came in and did it. Successful on the first try. After that, I was doing it ever since. I did that for about 7 months before I started home hemodialysis. If I go in the hospital, I put in the needles. If I go in-center, I do it. If you get a fistula, learn to put in your own needles!"

LeRoy Holmes Jr. – Started PD in 2003, did in-center HD
from 2004–2005, and then switched to short daily HD

You might be surprised at how many people we run into who get a fistula and then are shocked to find out that needles will be placed in it at each treatment! You need two needles for HD. One links to a tube that takes blood to the dialyzer (*arterial*). The other links to a tube that brings your blood back to you (*venous*). For many people on standard HD, getting the needles placed is the most stressful part of each treatment. Fear of someone new putting in the needles even keeps some people from ever leaving their home clinic. You can reduce your stress and feel less pain by putting in your *own* needles.

If you plan to do home HD or in-center self-care, learning to place your needles (*self-cannulation*) will be part of your training. Learning that skill ahead of time can get you over a hurdle and shorten your training time. You can learn to put in needles with your left hand if you are right handed, or vice versa. You need to be able to move your wrist, hand, and fingers. Some people who cannot see are still able to put in their own needles.

When someone else puts needles in, they can only feel the outside of your access. Since your access is in *your* arm or leg, you can feel the inside *and* the outside. Plus, each person may use a different angle to put the needles in—while you would use the same angle each time. Both of these factors give you a built-in edge *no one else* has, not even a nurse. **You are the *only person on earth* who can feel both ends of the needle—so you are likely to be your own best cannulator.**

Your access may last years longer if you put your own needles in, and this helps reduce your stress level. Remember those fistulas that lasted 30 years or more? They belong to people who put in their own needles.

Getting Past Needle Fear

Almost no one *likes* needles. But for some, needle phobia is much more than a minor fear: it's a terror that can scare you away from health care. And if you need dialysis, you may face needles often. Having needle fear does not mean that you are weak or childish. It's an involuntary response of your body—a *vasovagal reflex*—to having blood drawn, getting an injection, an injury, or even the sight of blood or *thought* of a needle. Needle fear is listed in the DSM-IV manual, the official book of psychiatric disorders, as a "specific phobia," called *Blood-Injection-Injury Type*.

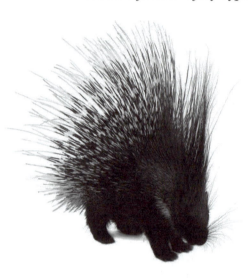

Here's how it works:

- First, due to fear, your heart beats faster and your blood pressure goes up.
- Then, your heart slows down, and your blood pressure falls. Your body puts out stress hormones. Your heart rhythms may change.
- You may become pale, sweaty, nauseous, light headed, dizzy, and may pass out.

Experts believe needle fear is part learned and part genetic.[25] Many people who have needle fear had a needle trauma in their past. About 4 out of 5 have a family member who has the same fear.[25] You may have both. Among the general public, at least 1 in 10 people are said to have needle fear.[25] But, the real number may be higher: one study found that more than a quarter of college students who did not give blood gave needle fear as a reason.[26] A study of people on dialysis found that *nearly half* said that needle phobia kept them from doing self-care treatments.[27] So, if you have this problem, you are not alone!

The degree of needle fear can vary. Some people can have blood drawn or get a vaccine without passing out if they look away and lie flat. Others are so fearful that they avoid *all* needles. They may even refuse care they need to live. If you need dialysis and are very afraid of needles, there are treatments that can help you.

Ways to Reduce Needle Fear

Since needle fear triggers the vasovagal reflex, treatment is based on stopping this reflex in its tracks—or training your body not to react. Here are some ways that have worked for others:

TIP: Bring more blood to your head – Lie flat, or tilt the chair so your legs are above your head when you get a needle stick.

- **Why it Can Work**: Fainting (or passing out) is your body's way of getting more blood to your brain when your blood pressure drops too low. If you lie flat or tilt the chair in advance, you can short-circuit this reflex so you don't pass out.

TIP: Tense your muscles – At the first sign of a problem, tighten your non-access arm, leg, and torso muscles for 10 or 20 seconds, until your face feels warm. Then slowly relax them—but not all the way—until the needle is in. Talk to your doctor before you try this. With his or her okay, practice this at home before you need to do it in the clinic.

■ **Why it Can Work**: Muscle tension can raise your blood pressure by forcing blood from your arms and legs into your brain. This can keep you from passing out—and help teach your body not to react to needles. In one case report of a pregnant woman, this worked so well that she was able to have many needles and procedures without passing out, even months later.[28] It has not been studied in people on dialysis.

TIP: Get Therapy – Ask your doctor or social worker to refer you to a therapist who can do desensitization treatments. These slowly expose you to your fears in a safe setting until they lose their power to scare you.

■ **Why it Can Work**: This type of treatment is used for phobias of all types—from spiders to heights. Needles are no different. NOTE: This may be paid for by Medicare or your insurance, since needle phobia is in DSM-IV. Medicare Part B covers "outpatient mental health services when performed by a qualified psychiatrist, a clinical psychologist, or a clinical social worker in the office or the patient's home, as an outpatient."

TIP: Avoid Needles – Choose a treatment like PD or transplant that doesn't use needles.

■ **Why it Can Work**: No needles, no vasovagal reflex. If you do HD, you need to know that using a catheter just to avoid needles may risk your life.[29] An HD catheter is much more prone to blood infections and blood clots than a fistula.

TIP: Numb the Pain – Use a pain killing cream or gel to numb the site. Please note that we are not talking about injecting lidocaine, which is often done in dialysis clinics. Why not? Two reasons:

1) Needles. We are trying to avoid them, so using one does not make sense.

2) Some nurses believe that either the needles or the lidocaine under the skin makes the skin tough and harder to place needles in down the road. There are no studies to confirm or deny this.

■ **Why it Can Work**: Pain is part of the reason for the fear. If you don't feel a needle, it may not trigger a vasovagal reflex.[25] A number of creams have lidocaine to numb the skin, plus something to carry it below the top layer of skin. It's best to use these products at least 60–90 minutes before you need them. Cover the spot with a thick coat of the cream or gel and protect it with a Tegaderm® dressing or self-sticking plastic wrap to keep it in place. All of these creams are messy and must be cleaned off very well before dialysis.

You do not need a doctor's prescription to buy most of these products, but we urge you to talk to your doctor before using them for dialysis. Some people are allergic to them. Read all package insert precautions before use.

EMLA® (AstraZeneca) is a cream or patch with 2.5% lidocaine and 2.5% prilocaine. It comes in 5 gram or 30 gram tubes; about 3 grams are used each time. If your doctor prescribes EMLA, Medicare pays for it under the dialysis bundle, and your clinic must provide it to you for free.

Topicaine is a 4% lidocaine gel often used to reduce pain during laser hair removal, tattoo removal, etc. It comes in a 10 gram tube for under $20, or a 113 gram tube for about $85. www.topicaine.com. (800) 677-9299 in the U.S. and Canada, or (561) 746-0365.

LMX-4 ("Ela-Max") is a 4% lidocaine cream. It comes in a 30 gram tube for about $50. www.skinstore.com/p-631-lmx-4.aspx is one online source.

NOTE: We list these products for information only. We do not endorse any product, nor do we benefit from them in any way. We do not offer any warranty, implied or inferred. Use them at your own risk.

TIP: Take Charge of Your Needles – Ask for training to put your dialysis needles in yourself.

- **Why it Can Work**: Knowledge fights fear. If you are not afraid, you won't trigger the reflex. Also, putting in your own needles distracts you from any pain you might feel—though you can also use a cream or gel. And, finally, when you are in charge of the needle, it is simply less scary than when someone else wields it.

There's no question that it can be hard to get up the nerve to put in your own needles. People who put in their own needles say that the intense focus they use to get the needles in distracts them from the pain! So, it hurts much less, which is a plus.

You can take baby steps to get used to the idea of putting in your own needles:

- Watch while someone else gets their needles put in.
- Next, watch while you get your own needles—even just a glance at first, if that's all you can do. Look for a bit longer at each treatment.
- Hold your sites at the end of treatment if you have not been doing that.
- Ask the staff if you can hold a needle to get used to how it feels in your hand.
- Think about using a topical cream or gel to numb the skin over your access.
- Ask the staff to teach you how to put your needles in.

How to Put in Needles

You can learn how to put in needles by having a staff person show you, step-by-step, what to do. It's more of an art than a science. There are few studies to guide how things are done. Each clinic does the steps a bit differently; it's best if you follow the steps the way your clinic or home training nurse prefers. Here are the basic steps:

1. **Gather your supplies**. You'll need needles, gauze pads, tape (you'll tear a number of pieces to length), a tourniquet, a cleanser for your access, clean gloves, alcohol wipes, Band-aids®, a sharps container (to dispose of used needles or syringes), etc. Reading glasses or a back-lit magnifier can help you see what you're doing. Have it all in one place, with tape pieces torn and ready to use, so things go faster. You may want to write a checklist of all the things you need, or your clinic may give you one.

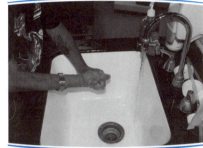

2. **Assess your access**. Feel for the *thrill* (buzzing vibration). Listen for the *bruit* (whooshing sound) with a stethoscope. Your thrill should feel the same from one day to the next, and your bruit should sound the same. A higher pitched bruit or weak thrill can mean a problem that needs to be fixed. Look for signs of infection, like pus, warmth, swelling, or redness. ***Never place a needle into an area of infection***—you could push germs into your bloodstream. If you see signs (or have a fever), call your training nurse. Don't place needles into spots that are flat or bulging. Choose your sites with care.

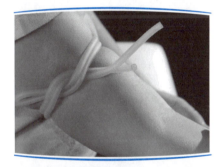

3. **Wash your hands & access**. Your clinic will teach you how to wash your wrists, hands, fingernails, and between your fingers, and how to clean off your access site. Use the soap or antibacterial product they suggest. Dry your hands well with paper towels, and use a paper towel to turn off the faucet. Put on gloves.

4. ***If you have a fistula***, **apply a tourniquet or blood pressure cuff**. A tourniquet helps you see your access, keeps the vessel from rolling, and tightens the skin so it is easier to put the needles in. The tourniquet should not be so tight that it causes pain or makes your fingers turn blue! Never use a tourniquet *during* dialysis. Tourniquets are not used for grafts.

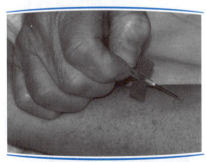

5. **Place the needles**. Your training nurse will teach you how to hold the needle and what angle to hold it at to reach your fistula or graft. In most cases, both needles will point toward your shoulder.[30] You'll grasp the wings of the needle and not touch it to anything but your cleansed skin. If the needle touches something else, throw it out in a sharps box and use a fresh one to avoid infection. Touch the needle to your skin and slowly press forward until it is in the vessel. You may feel a small "pop" when it is in place. Some clinics will have you attach a syringe to the needle with saline in it. Others will not. A "flashback" of blood in the syringe or at the hub of the needle once you hook it up will help you to see that you are in the right spot.

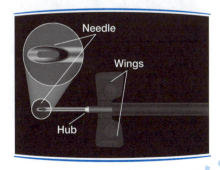

Needle

Wings

Hub

6. **Tape down the needles**. You'll learn how to place tape to hold the needles in place. For nocturnal home HD, you'll use extra tape, a Tegaderm® bandage, or a similar dressing to hold your needles and tubing safely in place all night.

7. **Troubleshoot**. If the arterial or venous pressures on the machine are high, or the needle hurts, it may be pulling against the wall of your access. Your training nurse will teach you how to gently move it to a better spot. You may need to tape a small gauze pad under it to help hold it in place at the right angle. *Never flip a needle!* Pulling a needle partway out and turning it over can scoop out some of the fragile lining of your access and cause damage. Nurses used to do this when needles had no "backeye" (slot). Now that they do, this should not be done.

8. **Remove the needles after treatment**. When your HD is done, you'll take off the tape, and slowly remove one needle at a time, putting pressure on the site *after* the needle is all the way out. (Pressing on the needle while it is coming out can cut your access.) When both needles are out, you'll hold your sites until the bleeding stops, then tape them or use a Band-Aid® as you were taught.

Using the Buttonhole Technique

When needles come out of your access after each treatment, they leave small holes. Over time, these holes can cause weak spots that can "balloon" out to form *aneurysms*. You may have seen "lumps and bumps" on a long-term access. These are what aneurysms look like. In a graft, there is only one way to try to prevent this: "rotating" needle sites by moving about a half-inch away from the last sites at each treatment. In a fistula, there are two ways to prevent aneurysms: rotate sites or use the *Buttonhole technique*.

The Buttonhole technique is also called "constant-site cannulation." It is not a device; it's a new way to put in HD needles. You choose one site for each needle and use those sites over and over. At each treatment, you put the needles in just the *same spots at just the same angle*. After 8–10 treatments or so, scar tissue will form around the needle into a tunnel—like a pierced earring hole—at each site. This scar tissue tract guides the needles into your fistula.[31] The two small holes next to each other look like the ones in a button, and gave the technique its name.

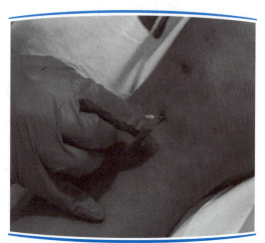

Once the scar tunnels form, you use special, blunt needles that are much less likely to hurt. The tunnels guide the needles into just the right spot. People who use the Buttonhole technique say it is less painful than using sharp needles at each HD treatment. Research shows that you are less likely to get aneurysms, too.[32]

To use the Buttonhole technique, you:

- **Gather your supplies**.
- **Assess your access**.
- **Wash your hands and access**.
- **Apply a tourniquet or blood pressure cuff**.

- **Remove the scabs from the last treatment**. Scabs can be removed in several ways, but moistening them first is most helpful. Use a sterile tweezers to remove the scabs. Don't use a needle, which can push pieces of the scab into your blood vessel and cause an infection. *Be very careful when removing the scab. A higher risk of infection is the only downside of the Buttonhole technique,[33] but infection can be prevented*.

- **Grasp the tubing just behind the needle hub and gently insert the blunt needles**. There should be no resistance when you slide the needle down the tunnel. You will need a little pressure to push the needle through the blood vessel wall. Never push hard to insert your needle. Call your training nurse for help if you run into a problem. Sometimes, you might need to use a sharp needle for one treatment.

- **Tape down the needles**.

- **Troubleshoot if you need to**.

Medisystems, which makes the blunt needles that are used for the Buttonhole technique, has a helpful brochure and a video so you can see this for yourself. You can view or download the brochure at: www.homedialysis.org/files/ADV223.pdf, and call 800-369-MEDI to order the video (*Constant-Site Cannulation with Buttonhole® Needles*).

Putting in your own needles is a vital self-care skill. It will help preserve your access so you can feel your best and have more control over your treatment. When you can put in your own needles, you *always* know that you have an expert cannulator close at hand.

HD Access: Graft

An *arteriovenous graft* links your own artery and vein with a piece of artificial vein. Most often, grafts are made of Teflon®, which—as in pots and pans—is non-stick so blood will flow freely through it. Like a fistula, a graft is under the skin. Unlike a fistula, the artificial vein will *not* self-heal after needles are placed in it, because it has no muscles of its own. For this reason, the Buttonhole technique *cannot* be used with a graft.

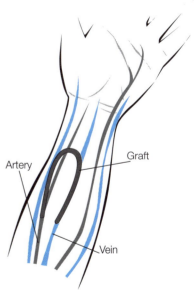

HD Graft

Over time, dialysis needles can cause holes in a graft that can make it prone to severe blood loss. Grafts should be replaced *at least every five years or so*, even if they look fine and seem to work. If you notice that your scabs after HD are starting to *protrude* (stand up), see a surgeon right away! This may mean that your graft is at risk of a rupture. Since Teflon is not native to your body, infection and blood clots are more likely with grafts than with fistulas. A study of 1,700 people on dialysis found that *the rate of infection was ten times higher in grafts than fistulas*, and the rate of blood clots was nearly triple.[34]

In most cases, grafts are placed in an arm. If you have no more access sites in your arms, a thigh or leg graft may be used. When these are not possible either, a "necklace" graft may be used. This type of graft goes from one side of the chest to the other in a large loop. This approach is very new, but in a small group of people on HD, almost 90% of these grafts were still working one year later.[35]

A new type of graft called a HeRO™ links an artery to the internal jugular vein in the chest, under the skin, using a piece of graft material. This device had less infection than an HD catheter.[36] One patient has had one for four and a half years now.[37] A HeRO can be an option for those who have no other access sites left.

Get an Early Start on a Graft

Even though a graft does not have to mature, it is still best to get one before you start dialysis. Grafts can also have surgical problems, and some time may be needed to make sure yours is working when you need it. It may take more than one try to get a working graft. Narrowing, called *stenosis*, is common at the sites where the artificial vein connects to your real veins, for example.

As you would for a fistula, choose a surgeon who has made many working grafts. If you have a graft that was placed without vessel mapping, you may be able to upgrade to a fistula when your graft needs to be replaced.

What to Expect

Graft surgery can be done with local or general anesthesia. After surgery, you will need someone to drive you home. Your arm will be swollen, and you'll need to take pain pills for a few days. A graft can be used for HD within a few weeks. You can expect that:

- **Your graft will vibrate**—this is called a *thrill*—and you will learn how to feel each day for this healthy sign. A graft with no thrill is a graft in trouble. *Tell your care team right away. Don't wait.* Call the emergency number you were given if your clinic is closed.

- **Your graft will have a sound you can hear through a stethoscope (called a *bruit*)**. If you have a stethoscope (you can buy one for $10 or so at a drugstore), you can listen to it. *If the sound gets higher in pitch—like a tea kettle ready to boil—or it stops, call the clinic or emergency number right away.*

- **Watch for any redness, swelling, drainage, or change in your graft after it heals, and call your care team**.

- **You will be told *not* to squeeze your graft arm** with elastic, a tight watch, or by carrying something across it. You don't want to compress the graft, it could cause damage to the vessel lining and cause narrowing down the road.

- **You may need ultrasound exams so any "mischief" can be detected early**, such as a narrowing in the vein or a poor blood flow. If found, steps must be taken right away to fix the problem, perhaps with surgery. It is much harder to fix a non-working graft than to step in and help one that has a problem but is still working. An X-ray dye test called a *venogram* may be used to pinpoint the trouble spot.

A mature graft will not enlarge, but you will have a scar, and a loop of artificial vein that may show under your skin. If it gets infected or needs repair, the scar will be bigger. As we said before about fistulas, we *all* have our scars. Some people on HD refuse to get a fistula or a graft, because they don't want scars. But chest catheters (see next page) leave scars, too—and they can be large and quite visible. Please don't avoid a fistula or graft for this reason, or you will surely be disappointed.

HD Access: Catheter

Most people on HD will use a central venous catheter (CVC) at some point. A CVC is a plastic tube placed by a surgeon into a large, central vein that feeds into the heart. Most often, this vein is in your neck or chest, and the tip of the catheter is in the heart. Sometimes a vein in the groin (*femoral*) is used for a short time.

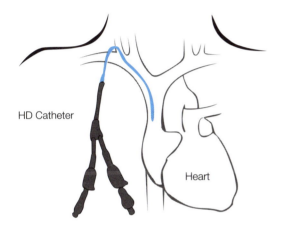

HD Catheter

Heart

Having a catheter in a central vein can cause narrowing, or *stenosis*, that can reduce blood flow to veins on that side of your body—so they can't be used for access in the future. Since you only have about 10 sites on your body where an HD access can be made, you don't want to lose any sites. **Narrowing is more likely if a catheter is placed in the *subclavian* vein. The KDOQI Clinical Practice Guidelines for Nephrology say that catheters should be placed in the *internal jugular (IJ) vein*.**

"Permcath" CVCs are inserted under the skin into a tunnel formed by a trocar tool. Your tissue grows around a plastic cuff to hold the catheter in place. Don't let the name fool you! CVCs are best used for only a short time, unless you have no other access options. Since a CVC goes from the outside world through your skin and into your bloodstream, it carries a vastly higher risk of infection. A study of more than 5,500 people on dialysis found that those who had a CVC were 54–70% more likely to die from *sepsis* (blood poisoning) than those who had a fistula.[29] Blood flow rates may be poor, which means you could get less dialysis. Catheters tend to clog up with *fibrin* (a protein that helps blood to clot) or blood clots, and may have to be replaced often.

You can hide an HD catheter under clothing, but it may cause a lump in a thin shirt or t-shirt. Not being able to get it wet means you may not shower or bathe as often as you might like, which could lead to hygiene concerns. Having a plastic tube coming out of your chest may be a constant reminder of your kidney failure in a way that a fistula or a graft— which are part of your body—are not. A catheter may be uncomfortable, too, and will also cause scars that can show in the neckline of a shirt.

Protect Your Access Arm!

From the day you are told that dialysis is looming at some time in your future, you need to protect your veins for an access. Each time you have blood drawn, an IV, or even a blood pressure taken, it can harm your veins so they can't be used for an access in the future. Don't let this happen to you!

Choose an arm early on; the one with the best veins. Your doctor can do this with vessel mapping. It's best if this is not the arm you use for writing. To protect your veins, *do not allow* blood draws, IV needles, injections, or blood pressure readings (unless your doctor says those are okay). These can be done on your other arm, or from your hand or foot instead. The staff may not know how vital it is for you to protect the blood vessels of that arm, so you will need to stand up for yourself. If you are in the hospital, insist that a sign be hung above your bed asking to protect that arm from any procedure. Only if there is *no other choice* should your future access arm be used.

What to Expect

A CVC can be placed in an operating room, a radiology suite, or a hospital bed. You may be given drugs to relax you and reduce pain. Placement takes about 15–30 minutes in most cases.

CVC placement must be checked by an X-ray to be sure it is in the right blood vessel. Ask the doctor what signs to watch out for to be sure your CVC is placed correctly. Once your CVC is in, be sure to ask how to care for it safely. You'll need to know:

- How to take a shower without getting the CVC wet
- How to change the dressing if you need to
- How to clamp the CVC if it starts to bleed

A CVC must be kept clean and dry all the time. There are devices to help you take a shower without getting it wet. Covercath™ and Covercath IV™ (www.covercath.com) are disposable sealed stick-on plastic bags that can be placed over the catheter to keep it dry. A Korshield (www.korshield.com) is a rubber and plastic poncho that can be reused. Each of these products is for showers, not for bathing or swimming. Medicare expects dialysis clinics to give these to you at no extra charge if your doctor prescribes them for you.

HD Catheters: Helpful Tips for Women

Bring along your bra (or draw an outline of it on your chest with a surgical marker). You can't wear your bra when the catheter is being placed. But having it handy will help the doctor avoid putting the catheter in an awkward spot.

If the CVC will be tunneled under the skin, find out where the exit site will be. Ask the doctor not to place the catheter exit near your nipple, as this can be uncomfortable and hard to keep a dressing on.

The weight of large breasts can pull a CVC out. Since you are lying down when the CVC is put in, if you have large breasts, remind the doctor so he or she will be extra careful with placement and taping.

Becoming an Expert

This chapter has explained the three main parts of dialysis: a membrane, dialysate, and an access. By getting up to speed on this core background, you are well on your way to becoming your own expert.

In the next few chapters, we'll go through the types of dialysis. And we'll do it in order of homeostasis. That is, we'll start with the treatment that is *least* like having healthy kidneys (standard in-center HD) and end with the one that is *most* like having healthy kidneys (nocturnal HD). Here's how it looks:

Standard In-center HD	Peritoneal Dialysis (PD)	Short Daily HD	Nocturnal HD
~15% kidney function	~15% kidney function	~15–17% kidney function	~30% kidney function
Chapter 6	Chapter 7	Chapter 8	Chapter 9

We encourage you to read ALL of the chapters about treatment options. But, if you want a quick overview, check out our lifestyle chart.

Your Lifestyle With Each Treatment Option

YOUR LIFESTYLE	Standard In-center HD	Peritoneal Dialysis	Short Daily HD	Nocturnal HD
Kidney Replacement	**15%** (Stage 5 CKD)	**15%** (Stage 5 CKD)	**15–17%** (Stage 5 CKD)	Up to **30%** (Stage 3 CKD)
Time Needed	**36 hrs/wk** for treatment, travel, recovery.	CAPD: **14 hrs/wk** APD: **63 hrs/wk** at night.	**16–26 hrs/wk**, plus time for supplies, clinic.	Up to **5 hrs/wk** during the day, plus up to **56** at night.
Needles	**Yes**, unless a catheter is used.	**No.**	**Yes**, unless a catheter is used.	**Yes**, unless a catheter is used.
Symptoms During Treatment	Muscle cramps, nausea, headaches may occur.	May feel full or stretched until you get used to PD.	Rare, because fluid removal is so gentle.	Rare, because fluid removal is so gentle.
Eating & Drinking	**Strict limits** on salt, potassium, phosphorus, fluid.	**Few to no limits**. Extra calories from sugar in PD fluid.	**Few to no limits**.	**Few to no limits**.
Medications	Many need 19—or more—pills a day.	Many need 10—or more—pills a day.	Fewer or no binders or blood pressure pills.	Fewer or no binders or blood pressure pills.
Working	Symptoms & schedule can make it hard to work.	**Work-friendly**. May have weight lifting limits.	**Work-friendly**.	**Work-friendly**.
Travel	Need to set up a slot at another clinic. Can take weeks or months.	Take PD with you. Have supplies shipped ahead in US.	Take machine with you. Have supplies shipped ahead in US.	Set up a slot or take your machine with you.
Body Image	Skin, teeth, hair issues may occur. Fistula, graft, or catheter issues.	PD catheter in chest or belly. May gain weight.	Better skin color. Fistula, graft, or catheter issues.	Better skin color. Fistula, graft, or catheter issues.
Intimacy	Loss of desire and/or ability may occur.	Fewer problems than standard in-center HD.	Improves with switch from standard in-center HD.	Best, other than transplant.
Fertility	Poor odds of having or fathering a child.	Poor odds of having or fathering a child.	Better odds with more HD.	Better odds with more HD.
Sleep	Many problems.	Many problems.	Better sleep.	Better sleep.
Survival	Worse than breast or prostate cancer.	About the same or a bit better than standard HD.	About the same as deceased donor transplant.	About the same as deceased donor transplant.

Standard In-Center Hemodialysis (HD)

For standard in-center HD, people go to a clinic for 3–5 hour treatments three times per week: Monday, Wednesday, and Friday or Tuesday, Thursday, and Saturday. In most states, technicians do the treatments. As of 2008, Medicare law requires techs to be certified, so they must pass at least a basic exam. Each clinic must have one registered nurse (RN) on hand for each shift, but most have more. Each clinic must also have a registered dietitian and a social worker with a master's degree. Some people do standard HD at home, with a care partner.

The 3 days per week schedule leaves a 2-day weekend with *no* treatment. "Days off" from HD may *seem* like a plus. Some kidney disease classes even use days off as a selling point for this option. But, a study looked at deaths among thousands of people on dialysis over a 20-year period. The researchers found that **the rate of sudden cardiac death—the leading cause of death on standard HD—was 50% higher on the day after the 2-day no-treatment weekend.**[1] Dr. Carl Kjellstrand, a well known nephrologist, calls the no-treatment weekend the "killer gap." He says that 10,000 people die in the U.S. each year who don't have to, solely because of this gap. So, we look at this schedule as a huge minus for you—*not* a plus.

Other leading doctors agree. A group of 15 nephrologists (who have written 2,900 research papers among them) held a cutting edge meeting on kidney failure at Harvard in April, 2009. Medical directors from the two largest U.S. dialysis companies were members of the group. After the meeting, all 15 doctors signed a letter to Medicare in June, 2009 to push for better treatment.[2] In it, they said:

"Thousands of lives have been saved through advancements, but the facts remain:
- *Mortality exceeds 20% per year*
- *At a cost of $34,000,000,000*
- *With less than 20% of patients rehabilitated*
- *And hospital costs per year exceed $20,000 per patient."*

They went on to say, *"The current formulas for prescribing and measuring the delivery of dialysis are insufficient. The original premises on which both the concept and the mathematics are based are incorrect. In addition, caregivers have relied on the formulaic approach rather than a full assessment of the individual patient. [This] one-size-fits-all approach has resulted in the "standard" dialysis prescription of thrice-weekly 3–4 hour dialysis treatments, which is inadequate therapy."*

We agree! Of all of the treatment options for kidney failure, standard in-center HD is the least able to maintain homeostasis. Because of this, it is likely to change your lifestyle more than any other treatment would. Let's say that healthy kidneys have 100% function. Dialysis should start when kidney function drops to 6–9% or so. Standard in-center HD keeps you just at the brink of stage 5 CKD. It gives you about **15%** of normal kidney function—at best![3] Before a treatment, your eGFR may be less than 5. After a treatment, it may reach 14–15—but in an hour or so, it is down to 11–12. Over the next 2 days, it drops back to 5, or as low as 3 after the 2-day gap. *The more HD you get, the better you can feel.*

How Standard In-Center HD Works

Choose a Clinic

In the U.S., we find that most people on dialysis seem to think that they were lucky enough to land at the only dialysis clinic in town. You would be amazed at how many had *no idea* that they had a choice—or that dialysis clinics differ. A lot. The quality of care—and even survival—can vary. Your choice of clinic can affect your life. If there is more than one dialysis clinic near you that your health plan covers, check them all out. You can learn more about this in Chapter 12.

Arrive Early

Once you choose a clinic, you will be given a time slot and asked to arrive 15 minutes before your treatment time. Wear comfortable, washable clothes—the same type each time, so your weight does not change due to what you wear. Most people who do standard in-center HD say they get cold. Tell the staff if this happens. Plan to bring a bag with warm socks, gloves, maybe a knit hat, and a small washable blanket or two. You may also want to bring things to keep you busy, like a book, magazine, crossword puzzle, handheld game (with sound turned off), bills to pay, letters to write, etc. Ask if you can use a cell phone or laptop computer. Some clinics allow these and some don't.

Someone should greet you when you come in, and on your first visit you will have forms to sign. Bring your insurance cards. Some waiting rooms in newer clinics have computers to help you learn more about kidney disease and its treatment. Other people in the waiting room may be able to tell you what to expect and how the clinic works. Beware of taking medical advice from others, though—their health problems may differ from yours.

What to Expect

When your chair is ready, a tech or nurse will bring you back to the treatment room. Other people will be getting their treatments at the same time. If you have a fistula or graft, you'll need to gently wash your access at a sink with a non-allergenic soap. Ask to be taught the right technique. You'll get on a scale to see how much excess water needs to be taken off. Then you'll go to your chair and the tech will take your blood pressure and pulse, and ask you about any symptoms you have been having, like itching, trouble breathing, headaches, stomach upset, vision or hearing changes, muscle cramps, or swelling. Be honest: your symptoms give your care team vital clues about how you're doing.

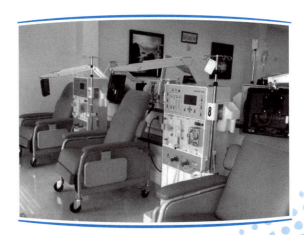

To protect you—and themselves—from infection, techs and nurses wear gloves, gowns, and face shields when they do a task that could expose them to blood. Staff must wash their hands with soap or an alcohol gel and put on clean gloves:

- When they enter and leave the clinic treatment area
- When they go from one person on dialysis to another
- When they go from one machine to another
- Before *and* after putting in dialysis needles, or touching a catheter or a wound
- Before *and* after touching someone who has a known infection
- After they touch any bodily fluid or mucous membrane (like the inside of the nose or mouth)
- Between tasks that involve different parts of the body
- After they take off their gloves

Watch to be sure the staff member working with you washes his or her hands and changes gloves before touching you. **Only let *clean* hands and gloves touch your access**. If you see that a staff person has not washed his or her hands, politely ask that he or she do so. This can be hard to do, but your health is at stake!

Always keep your dialysis access in plain view of the staff. Even if you are cold, your access needs to be visible at all times. When your blood flow rate is 500 mL/min, you would lose half a liter of blood per minute if the tubing came apart or a needle pulled out. Each year, between 40 and 136 people who do standard in-center HD die due to blood loss from a dislodged needle.[4] If you fell asleep, you might not notice—but the care team or the person in the next chair can help you if they can see your access. The Veteran's Administration now requires use of an alarm (called Redsense®) to alert the care team to blood loss.

Dry Weight

The tech will program your water removal, or *ultrafiltration* (UF) goal into the machine. How much will your UF goal be? That will depend on your "*dry weight*"—the medical guess of how much you would weigh if you *didn't* have lots of extra fluid in your bloodstream. (Water weighs 2.2 lbs. per liter.) This really is *always* a guess, because there is no good way to know for sure in a clinic setting. Medicine is part science and part art, and dry weight is a bit...arty. New technology, like body composition monitors, are in use in Europe and may come to the U.S.

One way to find out your dry weight is to pull off enough fluid that you get low blood pressure and muscle cramps—and then back off a bit the next time. Not a comfortable prospect. This is one reason to always wear the same type of clothes to each treatment. If your clothes are heavier, your tech could think that you gained more fluid weight and try to remove it. When you have a good appetite and gain "real" weight or feel ill and lose real weight, be sure to tell the tech, too. Your dry weight will need to be adjusted.

Some clinics have fluid sensors built into or added onto the machine. These sensors can tell when enough fluid has been removed, for a more comfortable treatment. In time, you can learn how much fluid you need to take off by how you feel before and after, and can tell the tech what your goal is.

Connecting to the Dialysis Machine

If you have a catheter, in most states a nurse must take off the dressing, check your skin at the exit site to be sure it is clean, dry, and not inflamed, clean the ports, and connect the dialysis needles and tubing to it.

For a fistula or graft, a tech or a nurse will clean your access, place the needles, connect them to the tubing,* and tape them in place. The tech will turn on the machine, and the blood pump will start to pull your blood into the tubing. The dialyzer will turn pink. About a cup of blood will be in the tubing and dialyzer at a time. Your blood will flow through the circuit and back to you over and over, getting a little bit cleaner with each pass.

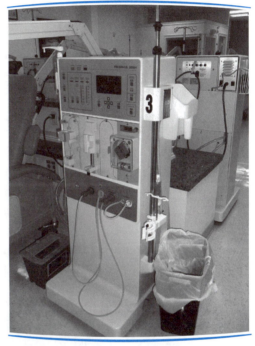

Some clinics *reuse* dialyzers. After each use, the filter is rinsed, filled with chemicals to kill germs, and rinsed again. The process can save money and cut down on landfill waste. But there is a risk of getting the wrong dialyzer back. Or, you could be exposed to toxic chemicals if the dialyzer is not rinsed well enough and tested for chemicals. Two people should check that the dialyzer is yours before a reused dialyzer is used for your treatment. You can and should be one of them.

Ask that your machine be turned toward you. This way, you can ask questions and learn more about your treatment, and then check the settings yourself. The machine has sensors and alarms to protect your safety. In time, you can learn what each of these alarms is by asking the tech or nurse.

*If you are afraid of needles, read our section on needle fear on page 46.

Finishing the Treatment

When your treatment is done, a bag of *saline* (salt water) will be used to rinse your blood out of the dialyzer and back to you, so you lose as little as possible. Then the tech will turn off the machine and take out the needles. **Do not let the tech press on the needles as they are being removed—this can cut the inside of your access**. If you have a fistula or graft, you or a staff person will need to hold (put pressure on) the needle sites *after* the needles are out to help seal them off and prevent bleeding. After they stop bleeding, a bandage will be put on the sites. When your blood pressure meets the clinic standards and you don't feel woozy, you can go.

At each treatment, you may get to sit in the same chair—or not. You may have the same staff person working with you—or not. If one staff person has a hard time putting the needles in your access, some clinics will let you choose who can do it. Others can't promise that you will get your choice. It is best if clinics choose a staff person on each shift who is an expert at putting needles into new fistulas or grafts, to reduce the chance of an error.

Taking Standard HD Home

Some people do standard HD, three times per week, at home. These days, with options that allow for better homeostasis, we don't suggest that anyone start to do standard HD at home. Still, as you will see at the end of this chapter, there was one study that found better survival at home than in a clinic—even with the same treatment schedule.[5] This may be because they really did longer treatments. Or, if they didn't feel well with a 2-day gap, they may have chosen to dialyze every other day.

Training

Until recently, people who did standard HD in-center did not get any type of training. Over time, from being through the process and seeing it done on others, they may have picked up a few facts. But one focus group participant we recall said, *"I've been on dialysis for 6 years, and don't know any more now than I did when I started."* We believe him. Since people tended to get just bits and pieces, it was hard to make sense of the information. Medicare rules changed in 2008. Now, your clinic is *required* to teach you about:

- **Types of vascular access**
- **Steps of the dialysis treatment and what to expect**
- **Your role in your treatment plan**
- **How to prevent infection**
- **All of your treatment options**
- **Rehabilitation—how to avoid or treat depression, stay active, and keep your job**

That said, dialysis clinics are very busy. Your best chance for finding out what you want to know is to ask. Be polite, and try to pose questions after everyone on your shift is on the machine (not while the staff is putting people on and taking them off). If you ask the right team member, you are more likely to get a correct answer:

- Ask the **dietitian** about what to eat and avoid, how much fluid you can have, and how your blood test results relate to what you eat and drink.

- Ask the **nurse** about your symptoms during and between treatments, and other treatment options.

- Ask the **social worker** about how to cope with the effects of kidney disease on your social, sex, work, and financial life.

- Ask the **technician** about how the dialysis machine works and what the alarms mean.

- Ask the **nephrologist** about your dialysis and drug prescriptions, and what to expect from your kidney disease in the future.

Like some people who do standard in-center HD, you might choose to learn how to do the treatments yourself in the clinic. This is called *in-center self-care*. In this case, the clinic would teach you how to set up, use, and check the machine, take vital signs, and perhaps put in your own needles. In effect, you become your own tech, but help is on hand if you don't have a care partner or don't want a machine and supplies in your home.

Why would you want to do this when the staff will do the treatments for you? When you do your HD yourself, you feel much more in control. And, you may be more willing to travel when you know it doesn't matter who is working at the clinic you visit, because you can put in your needles yourself. Or, as one person said, "*To the staff, dialysis is a job. For me, it's life!*"

Training for Standard HD at Home

Standard HD treatments are done on a standard machine, which needs complex water treatment equipment. Your home will need plumbing and wiring changes, which can be costly. Training tends to take 6–8 weeks, as you need to learn how to handle things like drops in blood pressure that cause cramps, nausea, headaches, and other problems. Many of the people we know of who were doing standard HD at home have switched to daily or nocturnal HD.

On the flip side, you have control over when to do your treatments, so they can be more work friendly. You can choose to run longer, so you can have a bit more to drink and perhaps a bit more phosphorus. If you can do treatments every other day, you can even get rid of the 2-day "killer gap" and feel quite a bit better. Knowing yourself, your body, and your access can keep you out of the hospital and save your life. Still, if you are doing or planning to do standard HD at home, we urge you to think about doing longer or more frequent HD. It's just more like having healthy kidneys.

Who Can Do Standard In-Center HD

In the U.S., standard in-center HD has been the "default" dialysis that 92% of people with kidney failure end up with, whether or not it suits their lives. Standard in-center HD may not be a good fit for most people who need to count on feeling well to work or care for loved ones, or who love spur of the moment travel. There are some medical or technical reasons why someone could not do HD:

- Infants and children may have trouble with the HD needles. Their veins are so small that it can be hard to get a good access. School-aged children or teens should be in school—not missing it for standard in-center HD treatments.

- People who have dementia or severe cognitive impairment may not know why they are at dialysis, or be able to sit for 4 hours. They may scream, moan, or pull out the needles. If they have an advance directive, their wishes should be honored—even if it means not starting dialysis. If no one knows what the person would want, a trial of dialysis could be done to see if physical or mental status improve. If not, dialysis may only extend life with more burdens and little quality. The doctor can explain the pros and cons of all options.

- Some clinics are not able to provide in-center care for people who use a ventilator. They may be able to train a person with a trach or ventilator for home dialysis—or train a loved one to do the treatments. Training can be done in the home.

- It can be difficult and costly to transport people to and from standard in-center HD who are morbidly obese and/or have lost a limb and can't walk. Home dialysis may be a better option.

Standard In-Center HD – Nancy's Story

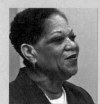 My name is Nancy L. Scott. I am a retired nurse and an ordained minister. I have been retired from healthcare since 1994.

I had a stroke in 1994 and a very successful recovery. In 1995, I began to enjoy my retirement. I began to travel and basically do anything I wanted. Life was great! Suddenly in March of 2004, I could not see! Everything looked white. I laid on my couch (my comfort zone) and tried to watch television. The people inside the television seemed to be stick figures. I tried to stand up and could not do it. Fortunately, my daughter, who had a key to my house, stopped by and took me to the emergency room. I could not imagine what was going on. My blood sugars were under control, as well as my blood pressure. The ER doctor took blood work and kept asking me about my kidneys. I kept asking him, why are you asking about my kidneys? You know the rest. I was in renal failure—end-stage renal disease.

I went to the ER on Saturday afternoon. Saturday evening, the nephrologist told me that I would be on dialysis by Monday morning. I lost it. I requested a second opinion and as many more opinions as I could get. Of course, early Monday morning, she inserted a catheter in my groin and I dialyzed shortly after. Believe it or not, the treatment was uneventful. But after it was over, I cried for the next 2 weeks as I went back and forth to the hospital. The nephrologist advised me about transplant. My daughter turned out to be a perfect match. Then I got a mammogram, which revealed that I had breast cancer. Double whammy! I received 33 treatments of radiation and oral chemo medicine that I would have to take for 5 years.

The hospital also told me I would have to go to a dialysis center after receiving treatments at the hospital for 6 months. I was livid! How could they send me to a center where the people giving the treatments were not even nurses? Of course, the techs were well trained and taught me the "education" of dialysis. I have chosen to stay with in-center dialysis because: 1) it gets me up in the morning (not allowing me to feel sorry for myself); 2) I do not to choose to live in cramped quarters with a machine and supplies at home; 3) Peritoneal dialysis is not my choice of modality because the solution is a sugar base, and I do not desire to return to diabetic medicines.

As I enter my 7th year of dialysis, positive things have happened. I am a 6-year breast cancer survivor and an advocate for dialysis patients. I joined an organization called Dialysis Patient Citizens. I am the President and Chair of the Education Committee. We help pass issues which affect dialysis patients. The Board is made up of mostly dialysis patients and healthcare givers. I have addressed Congress on several occasions, am on the Medical Review Board of The Renal Network, and am working toward a Master's degree in Health Care Administration.

I have started a support group in my area. I encourage patient self-care since I have been cannulating myself for 4 years. Knowledge is empowerment.

End-stage renal disease does not mean the end of your life, it just means the end of your kidney function. When diagnosed with this disease, educate yourself. Learn as much as you can so that you can have some type of control. NOTE: Nancy received a kidney transplant on May 4, 2011, and is doing well!

Living far away from a standard HD clinic is a concern, too. A study of nearly 21,000 people found that a longer travel time to a clinic (more than 15 minutes) was linked with a higher risk of death.[6] If you need to feel in control, it may be hard for you to do well on standard in-center HD. Privacy is also an issue for some, as a number of people all get their treatment in one room.

Your Lifestyle on Standard In-Center HD

We said in the intro of this book that your choice of a treatment option would affect every aspect of your lifestyle. In the case of standard in-center HD, here's how:

Time Commitment

Most standard HD treatments last 3–4 hours. All in all, your weekly time would look something like this:

Table 6-1: Time Commitment for Standard In-Center HD

Task	Time	Number of Treatments	Total
HD treatment	3–4 hours	3	9–12 hours
Travel to the clinic	20 min. (+)	3	1 hour
Waiting room time	20 min. (+)	3	1 hour
Travel home	20 min. (+)	3	1 hour
Recovery time to feel well again	7 hours	3	21 hours
			33–36 hours

If you have a fistula or graft and need to hold your sites, add an extra half hour or hour per week. One study found that people can feel weak and tired for up to 7 hours after a standard HD treatment.[7] (For some people it is less.) And, of course, your travel and parking time could be quite a bit longer than 20 minutes each way. For these reasons, even though the treatments may just be 3–4 hours each, standard HD may take from **33–36** hours per week or more—nearly as much as a full-time job, and much of it during the day. No wonder we say it isn't work friendly!

The timing of those treatments may or may not be a good fit for other things you need to do with your life. Those who are just starting at a clinic may be at the bottom of the totem pole. They may get the open time slots (such as 5 a.m. on Tuesdays, Thursdays, and Saturdays). If the time slot you are given doesn't suit your life, job, or ride to the clinic, ask if another slot is open. If not, in time, you may be able to change time slots and/or days. Or, there may be another clinic nearby that can give you a better time.

How You'll Feel During and After Treatment
Needles

For the most part, standard HD does not hurt. At the start of a treatment, you'll have needles placed if you have a fistula or graft. The needles may hurt for a few moments when they go in. Medication can be used to numb your skin, or if you have a fistula, the Buttonhole technique can make the needles nearly painless (see page 50).

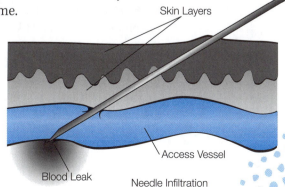

Skin Layers

Access Vessel

Blood Leak

Needle Infiltration

Sometimes a needle can *infiltrate*. It passes through the front *and* back wall of your fistula or graft, so blood leaks out into your tissues. This causes painful bruising, and can lead to a blood clot that could threaten your access. Learning to put in your own needles (see page 49) is the best way to prevent an infiltration and help your access last as long as possible.

Feeling Cold

During a treatment, you may feel cold, even though clinics must keep the room temperature comfortable for most people. Your blood comes back to you cooler than it started. The dialysate may be cool on purpose, because this reduces the chance that your blood pressure will drop.[8] The downside is, you are cold on the *inside*. Blankets, warm socks, and even a wool knit hat can help warm you up. A few clinics have warming lights over each chair or chairs with heated seats. Remember: *always* keep your access visible to the staff, even if you are cold.

Muscle Cramps, Headaches, Nausea and Vomiting

In chapter 3, we talked about homeostasis and water. **During dialysis, water is removed only from your blood**. Your *whole blood volume* is only about 5 liters. Most of the extra water in your body is *inside or between your cells*. If a treatment takes 3 liters of water out, your blood can get thick and sludgy. It takes time for water to shift out of the spaces between your cells and back into your blood. It takes even longer for water to then shift from your cells to the space between them. Fast, short dialysis three times a week just simply doesn't leave enough time for this balance to occur. So, you may be left with headaches, flu-like symptoms, and feeling washed out.

Water that is inside or between your cells—say, in your lungs or your ankles—can *only* be removed if a treatment lasts long enough. So, if you drink a Big Gulp, 32-ounce soda during a treatment, most of it will *not* be removed until your next treatment. Why not? Remember the three "spaces" in your body where water is: inside your cells, between your cells (*interstitium*), and in your bloodstream.

Taking water out of your blood with dialysis kicks off a chain reaction:

1. Water "waterfalls" from your interstitium into your blood, to keep your blood volume constant.
2. Your interstitium shrinks.
3. Water moves from inside your cells into your interstitium to keep it constant, too.

In the average person, this "waterfall," of water from one space to another, is limited to a maximum of 350–400 mL/hr. It takes time for water to shift in your body so all is in balance. If water is pulled out of your blood too fast during standard HD, the rest of the chain reaction can't keep up.

Have you ever felt like you were flattened by a steamroller after HD? Had severe, painful muscle cramps? Headaches? Vomited? Needed saline? Had to sleep for hours after a treatment? These are symptoms of taking off too much water too quickly. This strain can damage your heart.

How fast can the blood volume be replaced from the interstitium during a treatment? It depends on:

- Your blood protein (albumin) level
- How healthy your heart is
- How big or small you are
- How easy or hard it is for your smallest blood vessels (capillaries) to let water in or out

Let's say you are average sized, so you have a maximum rate of water removal (ultrafiltration rate, or UFR) of 350–400 mL/hour. Here's what would happen:

- You gain 1.6 kilos (3.5 lbs.) between standard in-center HD treatments. **Your UFR is less than 400 mL/hr.** Interstitial water can refill your blood as fast as HD removes it. Your blood volume *won't* drop. Your blood pressure will be stable. **You'll feel good.**

Or:

- You gain 3.2 kilos (7 lbs.) or more between treatments. **Your UFR is higher than 400 mL/hr.** Your interstitium can't keep up. Your blood volume *must* fall. The more your blood volume drops, the greater the chance that your blood pressure will drop, too. And, the older you are, the more likely it is that this will happen. **You'll feel awful.**

The more your UFR exceeds 400 mL/hr, the bigger the gap between water loss and refill. The bigger the gap, the higher the risk that your blood pressure will drop and you *will* feel awful. In the table below, you can see what happens when you need to remove a *lot* of water in a standard 4-hour HD session. A 3-hour session is even worse. If you make some urine, you can handle a bit more water removal. But, the more water you must remove, the higher your UFR has to be to fit into a 4 hour treatment.

Table 6-2: Four-hour dialysis treatments

HD Time (Hrs)	Water you gain in mL (Kg)	UFR rate	How fast water can refill your blood	Change in your blood volume	Chance of symptoms or BP drop
4	800 mL	200 mL/hr	200 mL/hr	0	0
4	1,600 mL	400 mL/hr	400 mL/hr	0	0
4	2,400 mL	600 mL/hr	400 mL/hr	-200 mL/hr	Small
4	3,200 mL	800 mL/hr	400 mL/hr	-400 mL/hr	Major
4	4,800 mL	1,200 mL/hr	400 mL/hr	-800 mL/hr	WILL HAPPEN

When we asked people in the U.S. how long their standard HD treatments are, some of their answers shocked us. We've heard of treatments as short as just 2 or 2.5 hours! And some people do standard HD only once or twice per week. We even know of one clinic that let people who filled out a survey end their treatments 15 minutes early—as if a shorter treatment was a reward. *We can't say strongly enough what a bad idea all of this is!* You might feel pretty good from day to day. Even so, when you get so little treatment, damage you can't see is building up in your heart and blood vessels, joints, nerves and bones. In the long-term this will harm you. And you *can* have a long-term.

In Japan and Europe, standard in-center HD treatments tend to be much longer than they are in the U.S.[9] In Australia, it is common for standard HD treatments to run 5 hours or so—vs. 3 or even less in the U.S. If standard in-center HD is your choice, having another hour or two for UFR can make a *huge* difference in how you feel—and how long you may live.

Symptoms to Report When You are On Dialysis

Sometimes things can go wrong at dialysis. The types of problems we will tell you about below are rare, but they can be serious. The machines have alarms, and the staff must be able to see you at all times. However, we want you to know so you can keep your wits about you and tell a staff person right away. Watch out for:[10]

Table 6-3: Symptoms to Report

Problem	What it Could Mean
■ In the first 15 minutes of treatment: Itching, chest or back pain, shortness of breath, low blood pressure, nausea	■ "First-use syndrome" – allergy to ethylene oxide, which is used to sterilize new dialyzers ■ Failure to rinse all of the chemicals out of a reused dialyzer ■ Use of a PAN membrane if you take ACE-inhibitors
■ Trouble breathing, itching, hives, burning, swelling, feeling anxious	■ Allergic reaction
■ Pain or tightness in the chest, sweating, trouble breathing	■ Angina
■ Skipped or missed heartbeats, slow or fast pulse	■ Heart rhythm changes
■ Headache, nausea, high blood pressure, feeling restless, confusion, blurred vision	■ Brain swelling due to "disequilibrium" (fluid shifts in the brain)
■ Chills, shaking, feeling cold, may have fever	■ Pyrogenic reaction to endotoxin in dialysate water— especially if a few people react at the same time
■ Bleeding around needles, longer than normal bleeding after a treatment	■ Too much heparin ■ Too many different people putting in the needles (forming a large hole) ■ Stenosis (narrowing) in the access

Missing Treatments

People whose blood pressure drops during standard HD often feel much better on the off-days between treatments. So, it may be tempting to skip a treatment and feel better longer, or to leave early and cut that last hour short. But when you only get 9–12 hours of treatment per week, missing just 10 minutes at each one adds up to almost nine missed treatments per year. One large study found that those who skip treatments are 30% more likely to die.[11]

If the last hour of treatment makes you feel wretched, it can be hard to imagine why you'd want to think about longer treatments. Wouldn't they just prolong the pain? No! Just the opposite. Since water removal is far more gentle, *longer treatments are much easier on you*. Longer treatments mean the last hour can feel like the first, with no blood pressure drops. Longer treatments can help you live longer, too. A study of 22,000 people on standard in-center HD in seven countries found that treatments that were *at least* 4 hours long were linked to a 30% better survival rate than shorter treatments. And, each *extra* 30 minutes beyond 4 hours was linked with a further 7% improvement in survival.[9]

Eating and Drinking

Food and fluid limits are a big challenge on standard in-center HD. Changing what you eat and drink is the hardest thing to do—and a common reason for conflict with the care team. One thing stands out: **the less HD you get, the more severe the limits will be, the harder it will be to follow them, and the more you will find yourself at loggerheads with the staff**. When you only get up to 12 hours or so of blood cleaning per week, you end up doing a good part of the work *yourself*. The idea is to reduce the build-up of wastes through strict limits on what you eat and drink. This means you must eat foods with less:

- **Fluids** – anything that is liquid at room temperature, like coffee, gravy, soup, and popsicles
- **Potassium** – like dried fruits, papayas, mangos, avocados, bananas, potatoes, tomatoes, and salt substitutes
- **Phosphorus** – like nuts and seeds, canned biscuits and baked goods, whole grains, dairy products, eggs, meats, dried beans, cola drinks, and chocolate
- **Salt (sodium)** – like lunch meats or bacon, canned foods, pickles, and boxed mixes

This list may not seem to leave many healthy options that you *can* eat. If you have diabetes, your choices are an even bigger challenge. In fact, dealing with thirst and the diet limits of standard in-center HD are one of the biggest struggles for many who use this option.

Making a mistake with potassium—like eating a big helping of raisins, tomatoes, guacamole, or mango avocado salad—can be fatal. Eating too much sodium will make you retain fluid, so your treatment is harder on you. Too much phosphorus will make you itch, and can cause bone disease down the road. If you choose standard in-center HD and you want a good life, *you must also choose to follow your diet and fluid limits*. If you can't do this, choose an option where you get more treatment so you can eat a more normal diet and drink more fluids.

The more you drink between treatments, the more water you will need to have removed at your next treatment. And the more water that is removed, the more thirsty you will be when the treatment is over. Taking off too much water, too fast, or needing broth, saline, or a sodium modelling program to bring your blood pressure up turns on the thirst drive in your brain, so you *need* to drink. This sets the scene for gaining too much fluid weight before your *next* treatment, a blood pressure surge...and so it goes on. It's a vicious cycle.

Food and Fluid Limits on Standard In-center HD

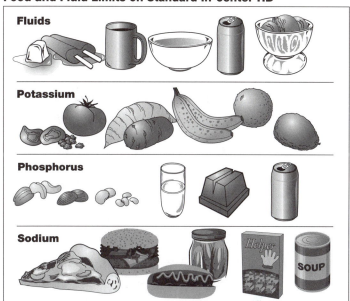

Fluids

Potassium

Phosphorus

Sodium

Potassium Too High? Read the Labels on Fresh Meat Products

A new study has found that "enhanced" meat and poultry and even fish are injected with enough potassium to be a problem for people whose kidneys don't work. Enhanced meats may have 28% more phosphorus and as much as twice the potassium of other fresh, raw meats. Read labels! Food makers don't have to tell you *what* has been injected,[12] but don't buy fresh meat with a label that says "Enhanced" or "Solution Added." Look for "phosphate" in the ingredient lists of other meats.

Dialysis clinics must have a dietitian who can work with you to design a food plan. Some will give you a long list of foods you are "never" to eat. Others will talk to you about your food likes and dislikes and help you make a plan that includes your favorites, at least some of the time. Portion size is key. A slice of tomato on a sandwich is not the same as a whole bowl of tomato soup. The good news is, if you choose to live with this meal plan, there are many sources of help for you. We list some resources for planning a standard in-center HD diet in Chapter 14.

Medications

Standard HD does not do a good job of keeping homeostasis because treatments are just three times per week, and they tend to be short. So, if you choose this treatment, you will need to take—and pay for—more meds than with any other treatment option. A recent study was done of 233 people on standard HD across the U.S.[13] Half had more than 19 pills to take and pay for each day; one in four had more than 25 pills per day. This was the highest burden of pill taking of *any* chronic disease—and with a strict fluid limit! Nor did all of these pills make people feel better: they rated their own physical function as low, which means they were at a much higher risk of hospital stays and death.[14-16]

These are some of the types of drugs that are common for people on standard HD:

- **Blood pressure pills** – to prevent damage to your heart and blood vessels. On standard HD, the "yo-yo" or "roller coaster" effect of taking off fluid only three days per week is very hard on the heart. Most people who do standard in-center HD need two or more types of blood pressure pills.
- **Cholesterol medications** – to help prevent damage to your heart.
- **Cinacalcet (Sensipar®)** – to help treat too-high levels of parathyroid hormone that can cause bone disease.
- **Erythropoiesis stimulating agents (ESAs)** – injections to treat anemia (a shortage of red blood cells) by making more red blood cells. Treating anemia can give you more energy.
- **Iron** – to provide the building blocks to make red blood cells.
- **Phosphate binders** – antacids or special drugs to help your body get rid of extra phosphorus that can cause itching and long-term bone problems. In the study of pills taken by people on standard in-center HD that we described above, half of the pills each day were binders.
- **Renal vitamins** – with kidney failure, "normal" vitamins could build up to toxic levels.
- **Vitamin D** – to help your body use calcium better and help avoid bone problems.

ESA Drugs and Safety

The U.S. Food and Drug Administration (FDA) has put a "Black Box Warning" on erythropoiesis stimulating agents, or ESAs.[17] ESAs are man-made forms of erythropoietin (EPO). Some research has suggested that if red blood cell levels reach near normal levels in people on dialysis who take these drugs, there may be a higher risk of heart attacks, strokes, and blood clots. In people with cancer, there is some concern that tumors may grow faster.

We are not sure these data are convincing. The study that worried the FDA most was not done in people on dialysis.[18] It was done in people who had kidney disease. One group was randomly assigned to a lower hemoglobin (Hb) level (10.5–11.0 g/dL). The other group was randomly assigned to a higher level (13.0–13.5 g/dL). Those in the higher Hb group had far more high blood pressure and heart bypass surgery at the *start* of the study. There were 4% more deaths in this group—but it was a sicker group to begin with. This study was also the only one that did not find higher quality of life in people whose Hb levels were higher, which calls the study methods into question. And we don't know whether it is a higher Hb itself—or higher doses of ESAs (often needed due to inflammation in the body)—that are the problem, if there even really is a problem.

Let's say the study is right and there really is a risk. Even so, living with a very low Hb is a bit like being a fish out of water. You may be aware of every breath you take. Simply going about your day can be a challenge. As some people on dialysis said when their Hb was low:[19]

"Oh, I can't do vacuuming. I used to love to vacuum. And to make a bed, my husband has to help me because I just don't have the energy to do it myself."

"Everything that I do is such an effort that I can't possibly do it. Even walking from the bedroom to the kitchen I rest after every two or three steps. I stop, because I don't have the strength to walk with. My quality of life has dropped so much that it's almost unbearable. I'm not able to do anything to help my wife."

"I used to wash all the windows in the house, for my wife, inside and out, and I would do that in about an hour, hour and a half. Got about 15 windows. So I wanted to help her the other day and I got finished with two windows and that was it, so that's my energy..."

We believe that if there is a trade-off to be made between length of life and quality of life, there is only one person who can decide: YOU. It's *your* life. Talk with your doctor about ESAs and the right dose for you.

Beware of blood transfusions, too. Each transfusion can help sensitize your blood to antibodies you receive. This could make it harder for you to get a kidney transplant.

Researchers are working on a new drug that would prompt your body to make its *own* EPO. If this drug makes it to market, it could one day lead to fewer limits on what your Hb level can be.

Working

It can be a challenge to keep a full-time job or even a part-time one when standard in-center HD takes as many as 36 hours out of your week. Even though about half of those who start dialysis each year in the U.S. are working-age (65 or under), fewer than one in four keep their jobs.[20] Dialysis clinics may offer standard HD in the evenings or early mornings. For some, this is work-friendly enough, if they feel pretty well. They may bring along a laptop and/or cell phone if the clinic lets them, and even do some work during their treatments.

For others, the "dialysis hangover" caused by taking off fluid just three times a week leaves them washed out, with flu-like symptoms after treatments, and fuzzy thinking all the time. Dialysis time slots can conflict with work hours. Symptoms, like fatigue, can make it hard to put in a full work day. The strict meal plan and fluid limits also makes it harder to eat business meals out. On average, people who do standard in-center HD spend about 12 days in the hospital each year, too, which means missing more work.[21] So, they may take disability.

Permanent vacation...no deadlines, no more boss. It may *sound* good. But most people don't know that Social Security Disability Insurance (SSDI) pays only about 35% of what you earn at work.[22] If your income is above average, SSDI may pay quite a bit less than 35%. To prevent fraud, even a good private disability plan will replace just 60% of work income (minus SSDI payments).[22] This means most people can earn much more money from work than they would get from disability.

Think about it: what would you have to give up if you had to live on just a third or even two-thirds of your income? Could you keep your home? Your car? Could you eat a meal out or take a trip? Could you help send your kids to college? Think long and hard before you decide to take disability. Once you do, it can be very hard to go back to work in the future. Most Americans qualify for Medicare to help pay for dialysis when their kidneys fail (see Chapter 11)—*even when they keep their jobs.*

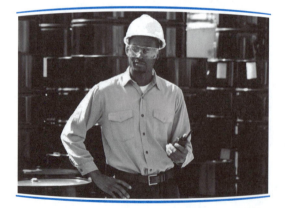

Research shows that people on dialysis who keep working feel better. They are more physically able, have less pain, and have better general health and energy.[23] And better physical functioning predicts fewer and shorter hospital stays—and a longer life.[15] Of course, people who feel better in the first place are more likely to work. But a job can also give you a sense of purpose, a place to be, an identity, and income—and those things may help keep you feeling good about yourself and your life. Perhaps for this reason, people on dialysis who keep their jobs are much less likely to be depressed.[24] And, they are also far *more* likely to have a health plan through work.[25]

An employer group health plan (EGHP) can help pay for treatment options and drugs Medicare may not cover. You may be better able to afford to follow your care plan—and to get a transplant if you want one—if you keep your job.

Travel

Travel on standard in-center HD for more than a night or two means making plans to get treatment at another clinic. This must be done weeks or even months ahead of when you want to travel. Your clinic's social worker or the company's travel service may need to help you. The new clinic will want your medical records, proof of immunization, insurance, etc. If the clinic is in a busy area, they may not have open slots for visitors. Or, the slot they do have may not be a good fit for your travel plans. Or, they may offer you a slot and have to cancel at the last minute, because they are full.

Once you get past these challenges—and we do know people who have—you can learn a lot by getting treatment at clinics in other states or countries. Rules that are hard and fast at one clinic may not be at another. The room may be set up in a new way. One new clinic in Miami even offers a spa setting, with soothing lights and music and personal "care coaches"—to people with good health plans.[26] You may come back with new ideas for ways to improve the care at your clinic (or bring new ideas to the clinic you visit).

Exercise

Many studies have found that doing exercise is key to feeling your best on standard in-center HD. Without it, you are more prone to muscle wasting. Toxins in your blood harm the tiny capillary blood vessels that bring oxygen to your muscles, so you may tire out faster.[27] Anemia adds to fatigue and makes you less willing to be active. Not eating enough protein to build muscles can also be part of the problem.[28] What all this means is that it may be hard to get up out of a chair, walk up a flight of stairs, or keep up with your kids or grandkids.

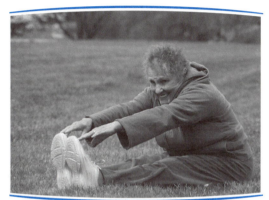

The less you do, the less you *can* do, so it's vital to find some way to move, bend, and use your muscles. That doesn't mean you have to do jumping jacks or run 5 miles a day. Anything from walking to dancing can help you build strength, flexibility, and stamina. Do something fun that you enjoy! People on standard in-center HD who stayed active had better physical and mental functioning than those who didn't.[29] And, among 792 people on standard in-center HD, those who had bigger biceps—a sign of more lean body mass— had better mental health and lived longer than those whose arm muscles were smaller.[30]

Exercise *during* dialysis can lead to better outcomes. A study from China found that peddling an exercise bike during HD helped people get a lot more treatment in the same amount of time.[31] In many people on standard in-center HD, the arteries are stiff, which can lead to heart problems. Using an exercise bike for 12 weeks helped reduce the signs of stiff arteries.[32] Can't pedal? Using a motor-driven bike to move your legs during treatments still removed more urea and phosphorus, and helped control blood pressure.[33] After 12 weeks of weight training during HD, 49 people had better muscle strength and size than those who didn't exercise.[34] And 12 weeks of yoga helped reduce pain and fatigue, improved sleep, and helped lower cholesterol—with no side effects.[35]

It is easy for researchers to study people while they are in an HD clinic. But you don't have to do exercise at HD to get its benefits. If you love to garden, like to shoot hoops, or live to square dance, go for it. Run your plan past your nephrologist first if you have not been active for a while. It's okay to take baby steps. If you are very out of shape, start out slow and build up slowly. Keep a log of your efforts so you can see progress, and reward yourself for doing well. Ask your doctor for a physical therapy referral if you can't do the kinds of things you'd like to do. Medicare covers some sessions.

You are *never* too old to benefit from exercise, either. People up to 96 years old gained muscle strength through weight lifting.[36] Weights can be as simple as soup cans—you don't have to go out and buy special gym equipment.

Talk to your doctor before starting a weight lifting program. People with kidney failure are at a higher risk for tendon rupture—with or without exercise.[37] Tendons are the silvery, fibrous tissues that attach muscle to bone (if you eat beef or chicken, you may have seen a tendon). Tendon rupture occurs when a tendon tears or pulls loose from the bone. The tendon must be fixed with surgery.

Body Image
Skin

Any type of dialysis or transplant can lead to concerns about body image. In Chapter 4 we covered some of the issues of hair loss and skin changes. Your skin is the largest organ of your body. It protects you from germs, helps you keep a constant temperature, and helps make active vitamin D. Standard in-center HD can affect your skin. *Hyperpigmentation*, or darker skin, may occur.[38] Or, your skin may look yellow.

In a survey of 363 people on standard in-center HD, 88% had some type of skin problem, from dry skin to pigment changes to tiny, cone shaped bumps on the upper arms.[39] Skin that blisters or tears easily can mean frequent wounds that are painful—and unsightly. Ask your doctor to refer you to a dermatologist if skin problems like this bother you. Since it can take months to get in to see a dermatologist, keep notes about the problem, and take photos if you can, to give him or her more to work with.

You can ease dry skin if you keep baths lukewarm and not too long—or stick to showers—and slather on a rich lotion after, while your skin is still damp. Talk to others on HD to see which lotions help them most, or ask your doctor or nurse for tips. Avoiding the sun may help keep skin from turning yellow. If it is yellow, getting more dialysis or a transplant can turn it back to a healthy shade again by cleaning your blood better.

Make an Anti-itch Skin Salve

This recipe was put together by the wife of someone on standard in-center HD. It helped him when no other product could. Maybe it will help you, too.

- 2 oz yarrow (flower and/or leaves), chopped
- 2 oz comfrey leaves, chopped
- 1 pint vegetable oil
- 1-1/4 oz beeswax
- 1000 IU Vitamin E (contents of 2 of the 500 IU capsules)

1. Combine herbs and vegetable oil in a crockpot.
2. Heat gently (do not boil) for 1–2 hours, stirring occasionally.
3. Strain and discard herbs. Pour the liquid back in the crock pot. Keeping it warm, add the beeswax and Vitamin E. Heat gently, stirring until the wax melts.
4. Turn off the crock pot and let the salve cool to room temperature. As it cools, it should be the consistency of peanut butter. If it is too runny, warm it again and add a little more beeswax.
5. Pour salve into a container with a lid.

This salve is good for itchy skin, skin rashes, diaper rash, burns, or use as a healing ointment.

Teeth

Keeping a healthy smile when you do standard HD can take extra effort. Healthy people make *a liter and a half* of saliva a day. Mainly water, saliva has enzymes to help digest starch. It helps wash bits of food away from your teeth. It makes your mouth more alkaline, so your teeth are less likely to decay from acid that forms when food breaks down. Minerals in saliva make tiny repairs to tooth enamel. Saliva moistens food so it's easier to swallow and less likely to scratch your throat. And, it lubricates and protects your tongue and the delicate tissues in your mouth. For all of these reasons, saliva is vital for healthy teeth and gums.

With a strict fluid limit from standard HD, you may make a lot less saliva. With less saliva to bathe your teeth, they are much more prone to decay. Less saliva can also lead to bad breath, gum disease, and tooth loss. In one study, the average number of teeth people on standard in-center HD had was 20—instead of the normal 32.[40] **Most transplant programs will require you to have healthy teeth and gums.**

Research has found that the closer a treatment can bring you to normal kidney function, the healthier your mouth may be:

- In a 2 year study, people who had kidney transplants made more saliva and had less dry mouth than those on standard in-center HD.[41]
- Much more gum disease was found in people on standard in-center HD than in a group on PD or a group who did not yet need dialysis.[42]
- People on standard in-center HD had more gum bleeding than those on PD—but both those on PD and HD had more tooth plaque than healthy people.[43]

Antibiotics at the Dentist

When you have your teeth cleaned, bacteria in pockets under the gum line may get into your bloodstream. These germs may stick to a dialysis fistula or graft and cause an infection. Some nephrologists prescribe antibiotics before a dental visit to help prevent a problem.

There are no controlled studies of whether this practice really does prevent access infections. This doesn't mean it won't work—just that we don't know for sure. Follow your doctor's advice about whether or not to take antibiotics before you have dental work.

For more than 50 years, the American Heart Association (AHA) has had guidelines for use of antibiotics at the dentist. They thought that bacteria from gum disease could reach the heart and lead to heart disease. Now, the AHA believes that only a very small number of people need antibiotics for this reason.[44] They are those who:

- Have an artificial heart valve
- Have had infectious heart disease
- Were born with heart disease
- Have had a heart transplant and now have a valve problem

If dry mouth is a problem for you, the Mayo Clinic suggests some things you can do:[45]

- Don't smoke, chew tobacco, or sleep with your mouth open. These habits can make dry mouth worse. Ask your doctor if you need help to quit smoking.
- Use a humidifier at night to moisten the air while you sleep.
- A number of prescription drugs can have dry mouth as a side effect. Ask your doctor or pharmacist to review your drugs for this. A drug change may help.
- Use sugar-free hard candy or gum to improve saliva flow.
- Avoid sugar: bathing your teeth in it raises your risk of tooth decay. Sticky foods like candy, dried fruit, or potato or corn chips (which stick to teeth once they are chewed) also cause problems.
- Some products are made to help dry mouth. Low-calorie Quench® Gum[46] comes in a variety of favors. Biotene® has a line of products that include mouthwash, toothpaste, mouth spray, gum, and more.[47]

It's no surprise to learn that brushing, flossing, and seeing a dentist for cleanings is key to keeping your teeth healthy. Getting small cavities filled can keep small problems from growing into big, costly ones.

Are you afraid of the dentist? Many people don't like to go to the dentist, but if fear keeps you from going at all, this can be treated. The **Dental Fear Central** website has information and even a dental fear support forum at: www.dentalfearcentral.org.

As with health insurance, many Americans don't have dental coverage. If you need dental work and can't afford it, talk to your social worker about local options:

- Some towns may have free or low cost dental clinics.
- Some dentists may do some free or low cost work, or offer a payment plan for costly repairs.
- Special credit cards are on the market to pay for dental or medical bills, even if you don't have a good credit rating.
- Discount cards can help reduce the cost of basic or more extensive dental work.
- If your area has a dental school or dental hygiene school, it can be a good source of high quality, low cost dental work. The students are supervised by teachers.
- A program through the Dental Lifeline Network called Donated Dental Services may be accepting applications in your state (www.nfdh.org/donated-dental-services-dds).

Intimacy

Standard in-center HD is known to affect sexual function. One study asked 117 men and women to compare their sex lives after starting standard in-center HD to their sex lives before. More than half had problems.[48] (The good news is, this means that nearly half did not.) What sorts of problems? Compared to healthy controls, 249 women with kidney failure in one study had less desire for sex. They were also less able to lubricate and reach orgasm. Not too surprisingly, then, they had more pain and were less satisfied with their sex lives. In this study, those who did standard in-center HD were more than five times more likely to have sexual problems than those who did PD.[49] Women were much more pleased with their sex lives after a kidney transplant.[50]

As early as 1975, a study noted that getting a kidney transplant brought back sexual interest in most men who'd been on standard HD.[51] This points out, again, how vital homeostasis is! Testosterone levels—which help drive arousal—tend to be below normal in men on standard in-center HD, perhaps due to a loss of zinc.[52] Like menopause in women, this is called *andropause* in men. Testosterone supplements help in many cases.[53-56] The dose may need to be higher than in men who don't have kidney failure.[57] Ask your doctor to refer you to an *endocrinologist* (hormone specialist), and *always ask* before you take any drug or over the counter supplement. Some can build up to toxic levels when your kidneys don't work.

Besides libido, men may be less able to get and keep an erection when they do standard in-center HD. If the blood vessels in the penis are in good shape, drugs like Viagra®, Cialis®, and Levitra® may help.[58] Diabetes or high blood pressure can damage the blood vessels so much that drugs won't help. If this is the case, a vacuum device or implantable penile prosthesis may make intercourse possible. One study had good results by giving men testosterone injections *and* Viagra.[59] If erectile dysfunction is a problem for you, don't wait to get help for it. One study found that over a number of years on standard in-center HD, changes occur to the smooth muscle in the penis. Collagen forms between nerve fibers where it doesn't belong.[60] It may be harder to help you if these types of changes occur.

Sex is never just about working genitals, and it's not just about intercourse. If you lose interest in sex, it may make your partner feel like he or she is less desirable to you. Money problems, stress, changing roles in your family, and never knowing how you may feel from one day to the next can take a toll in the bedroom. Feeling like a burden can make it hard to be intimate.

Communication with both your partner *and* your doctor is key. Talk things through with your partner. Hug. Hold hands. Make eye contact, and tell your partner that you appreciate him or her. Take a walk together, or plan a date. Dates don't have to cost extra money; they are a state of mind. Grocery shopping together or going to the library can be a date if you pay attention to each other and you call it a date. All of these little things can make a big difference. A counsellor or your clinic social worker may be able to help you talk about your sex life if it's hard for you to do so by yourselves.

Fertility

If you don't want a baby and you are of child bearing (or child fathering) age, you'll need to use birth control when you're sexually active. Pregnancy is much less likely on standard in-center HD, but it can happen.

If you do want a baby, it's vital to know that women may not release eggs while on standard in-center HD and men may not make normal levels of sperm.[61] A pregnancy in someone with kidney failure is high risk. You can improve the odds of having a healthy baby by getting as much dialysis as you can and treating anemia.[62] One woman had a healthy baby after doing in-center HD five times per week for three hours.[63] In a study of five women ages 31 to 37 on dialysis in Toronto, none got pregnant on standard in-center HD. Once they switched to nocturnal HD (three to six sessions per week of 6-8 hours at night), they had six live infants from seven pregnancies.[64] Another woman had a full-term baby after doing daily HD.[65] Other studies have also found that more dialysis during pregnancy can help achieve a healthy baby.[66, 67]

Sleep

All mammals sleep. But you may not know that sleep has also been found in fish, flies, and even worms.[68] Sleep fine-tunes your immune system and helps rebuild your nerves. And, many hormones are released during sleep.[69] We know that:

- **Poor sleep can hurt your heart**. In a study of women aged 55–65, having just three nights of 4 hours of sleep made cholesterol levels soar.[70]

- **Lack of sleep is linked to obesity**. In a study of 276 adults from Canada followed for 6 years, those who slept less than 7 hours—or more than 9—were much more likely to gain weight.[71]

- **Lack of sleep raises type 2 diabetes risk—in women**. A study of 1,336 men and 1,434 women ages 45–74 in Finland found that women who slept for less than 6 hours—or more than 8—had a much higher risk of developing diabetes. This was true regardless of their age, weight, smoking, physical activity, and use of sleeping pills.[72]

- **Being sleepy impairs driving**. Sleep loss slows reaction time, and raises the risk that a driver will cross the median line into oncoming traffic.[73]

- **Lack of sleep affects mood**. A large study in Sweden found that insomnia (trouble falling or staying asleep) was linked with depression and anxiety, and vice versa.[74]

- **Lost sleep, lost memories**. Memories "lock in" during sleep, so poor sleep can lead to poor memory.[75] (As we age, most of us become lighter sleepers—and more forgetful, too.)

Many people who do standard in-center HD report sleep problems. A study of 11,351 people on standard in-center HD asked if they felt sleepy during the day, felt drained or woke up at night. The researchers found that 49% had poor sleep quality—which was linked to lower quality of life and a 16% higher risk of death.[76] Pain[77] or itching[78] (which is a form of pain) made good sleep a challenge.

Changing the treatment shift time for standard in-center HD may help in some cases. One study found that people slept better if they dialyzed in the evening;[79] another found no change.[80] Using cooler dialysate (35°C instead of 37°C) helped people on HD sleep longer and better the night after a treatment.[81] Sleep apnea is much more common among people on standard in-center HD than in the general population. If water removal is poor, the tissues in the back of the throat can swell, causing poor sleep.

If you have trouble falling asleep, some non-medical tips that may help include:

- **Take a hot shower or bath before bed**. When your body cools off after you get out, it can help you sleep better.

- **Try aromatherapy**. Spritz your pillow with lavender or use a sleep mask filled with lavender flowers.

- **Write a to-do list.** If your brain won't shut off, it can help to let go of things you need to do tomorrow by writing them down.

- **Listen to soft music**. Keep the volume very low, and music may help you drift off.

- **Meditate to sleep**. Count each breath—in and out. Start from 1,000 and count backwards. If you like, you can do this to a favorite song. (Lullabyes work well for this.)

- **Set up a routine**. A series of I'm-going-to-sleep steps will help you wind down.

Benefits of Standard In-Center HD

Standard in-center HD is nearly always an option. Space permitting in a clinic, standard in-center HD is a backup for any other type of treatment. If you don't want to or can't do a home treatment, it is always there for you. Or, if you do a home treatment and you or your care partner need a break, you can do standard in-center HD.

Standard in-center HD equipment is not in your home, so you can keep your kidney failure apart from the rest of your life, and this is of value to some. You will also have a group of people—others on dialysis and the care team—that you will see three times a week, perhaps for years. If you like them, this can be a plus.

Problems or Complications of Standard In-Center HD

We've talked about homeostasis. Standard in-center HD does the poorest job of keeping homeostasis in your body, due to the schedule and the short treatments. In the short run, this can mean treatments that take off too much water too quickly, so your blood pressure drops and you feel awful on treatment days. In the long run, it can mean not enough wastes are removed, so you have a much higher risk of problems with nerve damage, heart failure, sexual and sleep problems, joint damage, and bone pain.

Feeling in control can be a challenge with standard in-center HD, but it can be done. Learning how to put in your own needles, and doing self-care treatments in the clinic give you an active role and help you protect yourself from mistakes. Learning as much as you can by reading, looking for information online, and asking questions can get you started.

Remember when you were in school, and some teachers were *passionate* about what they taught, while others were just marking time? This is true in all fields—healthcare, too. When you are in a clinic, you may like some of the staff—or people getting treatment—and not others. You'll see that some truly care about their work and want to help you feel your best. Others seem to view your treatment as just another task to get through. If you find there are staff who don't seem to care, see what you can do to get to know them better. People are people. Notice a tech's new haircut or ask about his or her weekend. In time, you might notice that you get better care. NOTE: *Clinics do not permit their staff to accept gifts, or loans of money, or see you outside of treatment time.* But most clinics are happy to hear when they do something well, not just when you have something to complain about.

If you are doing standard in-center HD now because you don't have other choices, your options may change over time. Perhaps you'll move. Get married. Get a health plan that covers a home helper. Find a roommate to help with home treatments. Maybe the rules will change for a clinic you want to go to. We know of people on dialysis who got home programs started at their clinics—maybe you could, too. You may not be in the same place a year or 2 or 5 years from now as you are today. Does life happen to you, or do you help make things happen for yourself? Your chances of being in a better place are improved if you make a *plan* to go to work, go back to school, or pursue some other goal. Your life is going by day by day. Talk with your social worker about goal setting, or visit **Kidney School** (www.kidneyschool.org) to learn and set goals at the same time.

Survival with Standard In-Center HD

We know some people in the U.S. who have lived for decades on standard in-center HD. How? They learned all they could, kept a positive attitude, and followed their treatment plans. No one lives for 20 or 30 years on standard in-center HD—or any other treatment for kidney failure—by accident. It takes *effort*, being vigilant, making sure people don't make mistakes with your care. It also helps to start young, be small in size, and not have uncontrolled diabetes. So, please keep all of that in mind when you look at the statistics we show you below. Statistics apply to *groups*, not to individuals. Just because the group figure may not look good does not mean that *your* outcome will be poor.

If dialysis was insurance, we'd be talking about "life expectancy." The United States Renal Data System (USRDS) tracks the outcomes of people with kidney failure in the U.S. And life expectancy is one figure the USRDS reports. Life expectancy is the number of years you can expect to live, based on how old you are now. The table below compares the general U.S. population to people on standard in-center HD, peritoneal dialysis (PD), or transplant.

Table 6-4: Survival with Standard In-center HD or PD

Age	US Population – Remaining Life Years	Remaining Life Years on Standard In-center HD or PD	Remaining Life Years with a Kidney Transplant
0-14	71.4	19.8	55.0
15-19	61.6	17.6	42.4
20-24	56.9	14.9	38.4
25-29	52.1	13.2	35.1
30-34	47.4	11.4	31.3
35-39	42.7	9.9	27.8
40-44	38.0	8.6	24.3
45-49	33.5	7.4	21.1
50-54	29.2	6.5	18.1
55-59	25.0	5.6	15.5
60-64	21.0	4.8	13.1
65-69	17.2	4.1	10.8
70-74	13.8	3.4	8.9
75-79	10.8	2.9	7.5
80-84	8.2	2.4	No data
85+	4.4	1.9	No data
Overall	25.2	5.9	16.4

Standard In-Center HD – Roberto's Story

The Beginning

In the early spring of 1980—on April 27, to be precise—I was taken to the hospital in Houston, Texas. Earlier in the day, I had gone to a local community clinic to obtain lab and test results from an extremely painful headache and what appeared to be jaundice.

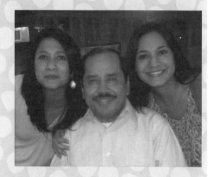

The doctor at the clinic said to my mother, "Take your child to the hospital immediately." He told my mother that I needed emergency dialysis. There was no delay. My kidneys had stopped working and my system was full of toxins that needed to be removed.

At the hospital, more tests were done to make sure that the reason I found myself there was true. I was 16 years old. Yes, I was very scared. Hospital staff tried to make me feel at ease, yet I understood that there was something wrong that was potentially deadly. How could this be? I was urinating a lot and often. Was not this enough proof that my kidneys were working?

A flood of questions popped into my young mind. Surely I had not done something that went against my belief in God. What had I eaten or drank? Are the doctors really telling me the truth? My kidneys would get well, given enough time, right? This began a belief that I would recover, but I should not take all of those drugs the doctors were giving me. At the time, I had to conform to the plan they were drawing for me.

On that first day at the hospital, I was told I would have my first dialysis. I did not know what the word meant. At the time, my mind could not comprehend the link to me. I was young, and all of the veins in my arms were small. Therefore, the doctors decided that I would need a temporary access. I had surgery on the bend of my left foot and the surgeon inserted an external plastic tube to give the dialysis technician a way to reach a larger blood volume. This was my temporary access while my right arm was being prepped for a fistula. As an emergency measure, the nephrologist inserted a catheter in my right groin, too. This catheter let them run my first 6 hour dialysis treatment.

I spent 3 months in the hospital, until I could recover and my blood work came down to normal levels. I still remember going to the dialysis clinic in my pajamas not knowing that I could dress in plain clothes! One day, my nephrologist assured me that it was ok to dress up. That day, I believe, was my graduation from the hospital setting and on to public life again.

My First Year

I soon realized that going to dialysis was something that made me feel inferior to other kids my own age. At the time I was beginning to get sick, I was in 10th grade. My calculus teacher doubted that I had enough knowledge to even pass on to the 11th grade. For a while, I could not play soccer, which I loved. Kids began to ask questions like, did I do drugs? They saw me with bandages or remnants of what looked like needle holes. I decided I should look as normal as possible so as not to attract any looks. I started a dress code, always wearing long sleeve shirts. What a difference!! I no longer attracted the looks nor the questions.

Then, of course, there was dialysis itself. My body needed to get used to having my blood being cleaned and having a few pounds of water being removed in a few hours. This process left me a little worn out at the beginning. My body began to feel stronger and stronger as the first year passed. I found that I could begin to play soccer again. I was able to graduate high school in the top 10 percentile.

My educational years

Convincing my mother of the need for me to leave home and go to the university was a job in itself. Three months before going to Texas A&M University (TAMU), 100 miles away, I began coaxing her. The day finally came when I had to leave. My parents by that time had already determined that I would be okay, but, they came to visit every now and then. I had an older brother at TAMU, which made it a little easier for me.

I found a dialysis center about 35 miles away from campus and began a trek in my 1971 Toyota Corolla, there and back, every other day during the week. I would leave campus around 5 p.m. and come back around midnight. My freshman and sophomore years were spent that way, until the medical director at my unit decided to open another unit just 15 miles away from campus, in Bryan, Texas. I had to dialyze 5 hours for the doctor to accept me as a patient. I now understand the need to dialyze at least 4 hours per treatment. In the middle of these things, there were times I doubted I would make it. But, then again, I knew that "all things work for good for them that love the Lord."

The Present

Thirty-one years later, I'm still doing hemodialysis in San Antonio, Texas! I graduated with a B.S. in computer science, and attended Arizona State University in the 1990s for a Masters of Science degree. I worked for American Express in Phoenix, Arizona for 2 ½ years, then was recruited to the Federal Reserve Bank in Richmond, Virginia, where I worked as a Systems Analyst. I moved back home to Houston, Texas where I began a consulting firm, Excel Publishing and Consulting, Inc.

Every dialysis session today is a mini vacation for me. At each 4 hour session, I give thanks to my nurses, technicians, and doctors for their care. Above all, I give thanks and praise to the Lord, for giving me this experience. For in it, I have learned what mercy means, in that, "*Wherefore in all things it behooved him to be made like unto his brethren, that he might be a merciful and faithful high priest in things pertaining to God, to make reconciliation for the sins of the people. For in that he himself hath suffered being tempted, he is able to succor them that are tempted.*" Heb 2:17,18.

Statistically, people are twice as likely to die in the first year on standard in-center HD than in later years. There are a number of reasons why some people who start treatment may be more likely to die:

- They are very old, with many health problems.
- They don't know enough about what to expect and how to prevent mistakes. As we said, eating too much potassium can be fatal. Getting an infection because someone did not wash his or her hands can be fatal.
- They use a catheter instead of a fistula or a graft.
- They are malnourished—many people who start treatment have not been eating enough protein.
- They are depressed, from loss of control and changing life roles.

Programs that pay close attention to these factors, especially in the first 90 days, have had a profound impact on survival. The Fresenius RightStart program had a 41% drop in the risk of death.[83] DaVita's IMPACT program has reported an 8% reduction.[84] Reading this book and learning to pay attention to how you feel and what you see going on around you can help as well.

"Adequacy": Don't Be Fooled!

If you do standard in-center HD, you'll hear the word "adequacy." The goal of standard in-center HD is to keep you from having uremia—symptoms of not getting enough dialysis. Uremia leads to many of the symptoms we talked about in Chapter 4, like:

- Itching
- Yellow skin tone
- Metallic taste in the mouth
- Nausea, vomiting
- Not being able to eat protein
- Having no energy

"Adequate" dialysis is a rock bottom minimum—not a target. It is the *least* possible amount of treatment that will keep you alive. People on standard in-center HD have told us that their clinics will say, "Your numbers are good, so we can shorten your time." They often think this is a plus. They get out of the clinic sooner. What's not to like?

If you've paid attention so far, you know that more treatment is better and you know why. "Adequacy" is based on removing a small amount of *just urea* from the blood and is measured at just one treatment per month. Urea was chosen because it is cheap and easy to measure—*not* because it is a key toxin. In fact, you could drink urea instead of coffee and it wouldn't harm you (though it would taste nasty). Urea is also a very small molecule that—unlike other molecules—freely moves between the three water spaces in the body (inside the cells, between the cells, and the bloodstream). This means that, unlike most other kidney wastes that can cause long-term harm, urea is very easy to remove. So, removing even a *lot* of urea does *not* mean you are getting good dialysis. In fact, back in 2003, one of the doctors who came up with the formula for Kt/V (see next section) co-wrote a paper that admits that phosphate removal with standard in-center HD is "inadequate."[85]

The "numbers" the clinic is talking about are URR or Kt/V:

- **URR** is the *urea reduction ratio*. This simple formula subtracts the amount of urea removed in a treatment from the amount you had before. It's a percent. So, if your urea level was 60 mg/dL before a treatment and 20 mg/dL after, then 60-20 = 40, and 40/60 = 67%. National guidelines have set the floor for URR at 65%.

- **Kt/V** is an extremely complex formula in which:
  - **K** is the amount of urea the dialyzer can remove.
  - **t** is the treatment time.
  - **V** is the volume of water in your body.

  How can we know the volume of water in your body? Good question. We can't, really, without putting you in a submersion tank. So, it's always a guess. How much urea does the dialyzer remove from blood? Another guess. The K, or clearance, figure is based on test tubes, not people. Even so, national guidelines have set a floor for your Kt/V of 1.2.

You have learned in this book that chronic dialysis started in Seattle in the 1960s. There were not enough machines to go around. Dr. Zbylut Twardowski—dialysis pioneer and inventer—wrote about what came next.[86] One effect of the short supply was that in the 1970s and 80s, clinics began to do shorter treatments so they could squeeze in more people.

Short treatments were said to be just as good as longer ones (based on short-term studies of people new to treatment who still had some kidney function). Larger dialyzers came out, which were said to make up for the shorter times. The rate of blood pressure drops during treatment began to rise. More blood pressure pills were needed. People gained more weight between treatments. The death rate from dialysis rose. And the Kt/V formula was developed for "adequacy." Its sole focus on urea took the focus away from other, much more vital factors like:

- How well people felt
- How many blood pressure pills they needed
- Whether they could work

Do you really want just "adequate" treatment? The bare minimum you need to drag yourself through your day? We think you might prefer *optimal* dialysis—treatments that would help you feel well from day to day, have energy, eat a "normal" diet, and be able to do things you enjoy. This can mean more work on your part. But might that trade-off be worth it?

Survival on Standard Home HD
Survival on standard HD does seem to be far better by just being home, even *with* the 2-day "killer gap." A study matched each person trained for standard home HD at one center between 1970 and 1995 (103 people) with someone who did standard HD in the center.[5] Pairs were matched based on age, gender, how long they had been on dialysis, and what caused their kidney failure. About half of the people in each group received a transplant. But the people who did standard HD at home were in the hospital less. They needed fewer surgeries. And in Table 6-5, you can see that at each stage, survival was about 50% better at home:

Table 6-5: Survival on Standard HD at Home vs In-Center

Standard HD Location	5 Year Survival	10 Year Survival	20 Year Survival
Home	93%	72%	34%
In-Center	64%	48%	23%

Why did the home HD people do so much better? We don't know for sure, but here are some reasons that might explain it:

- At home, it is easy to do *longer and/or more frequent treatments* that do a better job of removing fluid and middle molecules
- Home dialyzors know more about their treatment, so they are better able to prevent fatal mistakes
- Accesses do better with just one person putting needles in
- People at home are not exposed to the germs of a whole clinic, three times per week

In Chapter 3, we talked about wastes that *do* matter—things like p-cresol and beta-2 microglobulin. Standard HD in a center does not do a good job of removing these, and standard HD at home may be only a bit better. Don't be fooled by "the numbers" on standard HD. *Ask your doctor to prescribe longer treatments.* The DOPPS study with 22,000 people showed 30% better survival when standard HD treatments were *at least* 4 hours long.[9] You have a good chance of getting more time if you ask for it. And follow your treatment plan—diet, fluids, meds, and dialysis—as closely as you can—to have the best chance of feeling well. When you feel better with more dialysis, tell others at your clinic! You could help them improve their quality of life and live longer, too.

Wrapping Up Standard In-center HD

Now you've learned about the ups and downs of the treatment option 92% of people in the U.S. use when their kidneys fail. You won't be surprised to learn that if we had our way, standard in-center HD would be a treatment of *last* resort—not first, as it is now. We only have the standard in-center HD schedule due to a historical accident. In the early 1960s when chronic dialysis first started in Seattle, it was very costly. Without enough machines to go around, doctors experimented. With one day of treatment per week, people died. Two days: they died. But with 3 days, people lived. And, with money tight, they never tried 4 or 5 or 6 days. In 1972, when Medicare began to pay for dialysis, they kept to the three times per week schedule. *But Medicare never said how long those treatments had to be.* In the 1960s, treatments were 5-8 hours long. By the 1980s, some were as short as 2 hours.

It's great to have standard in-center HD as a backup, but we hope it isn't your first choice, or at least not for long. If it is, do everything in your power to stay in control, take an active role in your care, follow your treatment plan, and get as much treatment as you can. You'll feel best that way. Read on to learn about PD.

Peritoneal Dialysis (PD)

Peritoneal Dialysis (PD) is a self-care treatment you do at home. Learning to do your own treatments puts you in charge of your life. It gives you back some of the control you lost when you found out you had kidney failure. And, feeling in control boosts quality of life for people on dialysis.[1-3]

In the U.S., 43.7% of people did not even see a nephrologist before their kidneys failed and they had to start dialysis right away. Another 25% had less than 1 year's notice that they would need dialysis.[4] If you need dialysis in a hurry, PD can be a far better choice than having an HD catheter put in and starting treatment in a clinic. A PD catheter can be placed and used the same day (you do the treatment lying down) with no added risk.[5] Even if you only use it for a short time, PD can buy you a chance to keep your job, choose a different treatment, or get a transplant. Or, some people have used PD for years.

Like standard in-center HD, PD replaces about 15% of kidney function. Since fluid removal is much more gentle, PD does not have the roller coaster ups-and-downs of standard in-center HD. It is _much_ easier on your heart. But the waste removal of PD is about the same as standard in-center HD. So, the risk of long-term problems with nerves, joints, and bones, and the rates of survival are about the same, too.

How PD Works

The membrane that cleans your blood is the sac that lines the inside of your abdomen: your _peritoneum._ Your peritoneum is a shiny membrane layer that starts under your diaphragm and stretches down into the pelvis where your bladder and lower bowel are. It holds all of your loops of bowel, liver, spleen, and kidneys. The peritoneum is one cell layer thick. Under it is a layer of tissue rich in small capillary blood vessels that can be used to clean your blood.

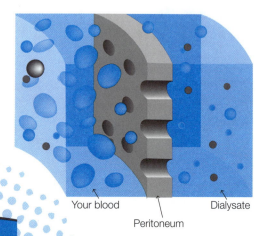

Your blood • Peritoneum • Dialysate

The access for PD is a _catheter_ (tube) placed in your abdomen or chest[6] by a surgeon. You use the catheter to put sterile _dialysate_ (cleansing fluid) into your belly. After a few hours of "dwell" time—while you go about your day—wastes and excess fluid in your blood flow through tiny blood vessels in your peritoneum into the dialysate. Then, you drain out the used dialysate and put in a clean bag. This process is called an _exchange._ Since your blood never goes out of your body, no needles are used for PD.

In this figure, your peritoneum is shown in the middle. On the left is your bloodstream. Blood cells and some proteins are too large to pass through the pores (holes) in your peritoneum. On the right, you can see dialysate, with wastes and water flowing into it.

PD By Hand

There are two main ways to do PD. One way is to do exchanges by hand—at breakfast, lunch, dinner, and bedtime. Each one takes about 30 minutes. This is called **continuous *ambulatory* (walking around) PD**, or **CAPD**. Most people train to do CAPD first. People who like CAPD say that once they get used to it, the exchanges are a lot like brushing your teeth: you do them without having to think much about it. As long as you do all of your exchanges each day, the timing can be shifted around a bit to fit in work, shopping, doctor visits, etc.

CAPD fluid bags come in sizes:

- **500 mL (about a pint or ½ liter)**
- **1,000 mL (about a quart, or ½ liter)**
- **2,000 mL (2 liters)**
- **2,500 mL (2½ liters)**
- **3,000 mL (3 liters)**

This means that the volume of fluid you use for CAPD will always be 500 mL or more. At first, you will start with smaller bags. In time, your doctor will likely have you start to use larger ones.

PD with a Cycler Machine

The other option is to do PD exchanges with a cycler machine at night while you sleep. This is called **continuous cycling PD (CCPD)** or **automated PD (APD)**. In the U.S., most people who do PD use a cycler. A *meta-analysis* (study of studies) found that PD with a cycler seems to have fewer infections and allows more time for work, family, and social life than doing PD by hand.[7]

Even with a cycler, you might still do some exchanges by hand if you like to do weekend travel or the power goes out. Some people end up doing an exchange or two by hand each day *and* using a cycler at night to feel their best.

APD can be easily tailored to fit your body and your lifestyle:[8]

- **With APD, the cycler can be very precise**. Changes in PD fluid volume can be as small as just 100 mL—less than half a cup. Over time, there is often a drop in the amount of kidney function you have left. If that happens, your doctor can prescribe a *little* more PD at a time, instead of a whole half-liter.

- **Your doctor can prescribe a different fill volume at night, when you lie flat, than in the day when you are up and about**. This lets you get more PD without feeling "stretched." Using less fluid for a while can also help if you are healing from a hernia repair.

- **APD does *not* need to last longer than 8 or 9 hours or so at night**. Rather than staying on a cycler for 10 to 12 hours, you may be able to use the cycler for 6-9 hours. Then, talk to your doctor about adding a mid-day exchange at a work lunch break, in the afternoon (after school for a child), or even after supper—whenever it fits best into your day.

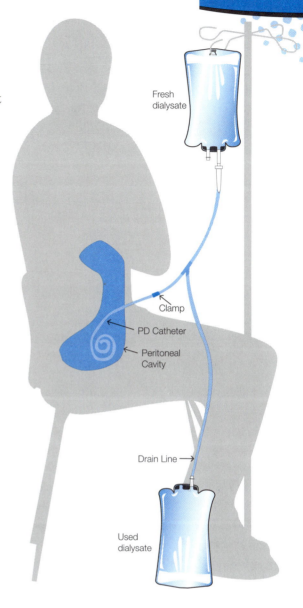

Fresh dialysate

Clamp

PD Catheter

Peritoneal Cavity

Drain Line

Used dialysate

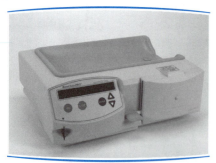

Baxter HomeChoice™ PD Cycler
Photo permission of Baxter Healthcare Corporation.

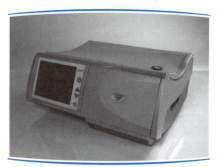

Fresenius Liberty® PD Cycler
Photo permission of Fresenius Medical Care – North America

Choosing the Right Type of PD for You

Which type of PD will work best for you? Until you start to do PD, there is no way to tell how well it will take wastes and water out of your blood. Your body is unique. After a few weeks on CAPD, a *peritoneal equilibrium test* (PET) can suggest how long the PD fluid should stay in your belly to give you the best results.

A PET measures how well *your* peritoneum removes wastes and water. To do the test, you'll come into the clinic in the morning. Plan to be there for 4 hours or more. Here are the steps in the standard PET (Your clinic may do a PET in a different way.):

1. Drain out last night's PD fluid.

2. Lie down and fill with two liters of 2.5% dextrose fluid at 200 mL/min. for 10 minutes. Each 2 minutes, you'll roll from side to side to be sure the fluid is well mixed.

3. As soon as all of the fluid is in, you'll drain out 200 mL, and a 10 mL sample will be taken. The rest will be put back into your belly.

4. You'll walk or move around for 2 hours while the fluid dwells. Then, a second sample of drain fluid will be taken, and a blood sample will be drawn.

5. After 2 more hours of dwell time, you'll sit up or stand to drain. The drain volume will be checked and another sample of the drain fluid will be taken.

6. Each of the drain fluid samples and your blood will be tested to see how much glucose and creatinine (a waste removed by dialysis) are present.

What PET Results Mean to You

A PET will show if your peritoneum has a high, average, or low transport (waste removal) rate. The test looks at your drain volume, how much dextrose is left in the fluid sample, and how much creatinine is in your drain fluid vs. your blood.

The table below, adapted from the UK National Kidney Foundation,[9] helps show you what each level means in terms of the type of PD that is the best fit for you:

Table 7-1: Choosing the Right Type of PD for You

Transport Rate	Waste Removal	Water Removal	Your Best PD Match
High	Fast	Poor	**APD**–Short dwells and frequent exchanges
Average	Okay	Okay	**APD** or **CAPD**
Low	Slow	Good	**CAPD** or **Reverse APD**

As you can see, if you are a **high transporter**, your best match is a cycler (automated PD, or APD). Short, fast exchanges will help keep you from absorbing too much PD fluid or dextrose.

If you are a **low transporter**, it may be best if you do exchanges by hand (CAPD) and space them out well so you have lots of dwell time to remove wastes. Or, **reverse APD** may work well for you: instead of doing a few fast exchanges at night with a cycler, your doctor might prescribe two slow 4 or 4.5 hour exchanges plus two daytime exchanges spaced 7 or 8 hours apart. This would let you use a cycler and do fewer daytime exchanges than if you just did CAPD.

If you are an **average transporter**, you can choose which type of PD you'd prefer—either should work for you.

PD Training

PD is easy to learn and to do. In most cases, you can learn it in a week or two. You don't need a partner for PD, unless you can't lift the bags of dialysate or make the tubing connections by yourself. If your hands or eyes don't work well, you may prefer to do PD with a helper, but training programs don't require you to have one. Your PD training nurse will teach you how to:

- Set up an exchange room
- Wash your hands
- Care for your catheter and your *exit site* (where the catheter comes out of your body)
- Do an exchange
- Choose which dialysate to use
- Store and order your supplies
- Keep treatment logs
- Take your blood pressure, pulse, temperature, and weight
- Follow your diet and fluid limits
- Recognize and report any problems

A PD nurse will be on-call 24 hours a day if you need help. You will not do exchanges alone until both you and your nurse are *confident* that you can do all of the steps safely. You will have a home visit, so your care team can learn how your house is set up, help you to choose a room for exchanges, and be better able to help you solve problems down the road if you need help.

Who Can Do PD

Until 2008, when Medicare started to require that people be told about all of their options, those who were white, working, had at least a high school education, and were married were more likely to be told about PD.[10] But when people were educated about *all* of the options, one study found that 45% of 5,065 patients said they'd prefer PD.[11]

Most people *don't* know about all of the options before they start treatment. In a study of people new to dialysis in California, lack of education about options was the main reason why they did not choose home treatments: 66% did not know about PD, 88% did not know about home HD, and 74% did not know about transplant.[12]

The truth is, *most* people can do PD. You may not be able to if you have had multiple or complex abdominal surgeries (simple surgeries like hernia repair, a kidney transplant, or a Caesarean section are not a problem). You'll need a clean, dry place in your home with enough room to store a month's worth of supplies. This can be a large closet, a garage (if it always stays above freezing), or along a wall.

You'll need to go to the clinic once a month for blood tests and once a month to meet with your care team. You'll need to keep pets out of the room and control the air flow when you do an exchange. And, you'll need to care for your catheter and do each exchange with care to avoid infection.

Most people can do PD even if they are:

- **Only able to use one arm** – You need to be able to connect your catheter to the PD bags. But you don't need two hands to do it. With an assist device to hold the tubing, you can safely connect with one hand. More than 10 years ago, a clinic in Indiana found a way to help a patient use the Baxter Ultrabag system with one hand. Baxter engineers used their idea to make the EZ-Aide Assist Device®.[13] Your PD nurse can order this today—it's Baxter item number 5C4505.[14] Your clinic uses Fresenius PD supplies? No problem. The stay·safe® system has just one connection. A control dial guides you through the steps of the exchange. A patient who had only the use of his left arm was able to do PD by himself using the stay·safe.[15] This two bag system is easy to learn and use.[16]

- **Not able to see well** – You are not alone if you want to do PD and you can't see well, or at all. More than 40% of people on dialysis in the U.S. have diabetes, which can cause vision loss along with kidney damage. At this time, PD cyclers don't talk. We believe talking screens may come soon. Meanwhile, blind people have been able to use CAPD, where exchanges are done by hand. In fact, in a British study, blind people on PD had less peritonitis (infection) and *fewer* PD problems than sighted ones![17] In one case study, a blind woman who has kidney failure wanted to do PD so she could care for her young daughter. With a talking scale and blood pressure cuff, and the Fresenius Premier™ Plus double-bag system, she learned to do PD. She was taught that abdominal pain might mean peritonitis and she should call her nurse.[18] This same system has been used in Canada with success to train blind people to do PD.[19]

  In Poland, a program was started to train blind people to do CAPD, also using a two bag system. They had good results, with just one case of peritonitis per 28 months of PD.[20] A 10-year study found that keys to survival and PD success in blind people were:

  - Motivation
  - Acceptance of health problems
  - Family support
  - Staff who were willing to train people who are blind to do PD

  In this study as well, blind people did just as well as sighted ones.[21] You may have to search for a clinic that will train you for PD. Your nurse will need to feel that you can learn the steps and do them in order without risking infection. Using a tape recorder to take notes during training can help you recall the steps.

- **Hearing impaired** – It's no problem at all to do CAPD if you can't hear. But can you use a cycler? With a bit of creativity, the answer is yes. A clinic in Philadelphia changed the standard alarm on a PD cycler from a beep to a vibration. They used a Sonic Alert Wake Up Alarm with a Sonic Alert Super Shaker™ Bed Vibrator.[22] With a vibrator pad under the pillow or mattress, you can feel the alarm and wake up to take action.

■ **In their 80s or 90s** – Age alone should not keep you from doing PD. PD can help you stay more independent, and may help you keep your remaining kidney function longer.[23] A review of studies found that most older people had the hand-eye and thinking skills needed to do PD. Plus, they tended to follow their treatment plans very closely.[24] They did not have any more PD problems than younger people.[25] Other studies of people on PD in their 80s[26] and 90s[27] found few PD-related problems—and just one hospital stay per 2.5 patient years (not just for dialysis). While most of these seniors did need some help at home, the authors say PD is safe for older people.[26] If you live alone, you'd need to be able to lift the bags onto the cycler or an IV pole for CAPD. Joint pain in your hands or nerve damage so that you can't feel your fingers would make it hard to do PD without help.

■ **Overweight or Obese** – These days, a lot of us are overweight, and that includes people with kidney failure. In fact, since so much kidney failure is caused by type 2 diabetes, *many* people on dialysis are overweight. Yes, you can do PD, but you need to be careful. PD catheter infections are more likely. Using a *presternal* PD catheter— placed in the chest instead of the belly—can help reduce this risk.[28] Overweight people also have a much higher risk for peritonitis, though the reasons why are not clear.[29]

A 2-year study of heavy vs. normal weight people on PD found no survival differences.[30] But, an Australian study looked at 9,679 people on PD at four levels of weight:

1. **Obese** (body mass index (BMI) >30)
2. **Overweight** (BMI of 25–29.9)
3. **Normal** (BMI of 20–24.9)
4. **Underweight** (BMI <20)

The authors found lower survival in obese people on PD and suggested close follow up to be sure all is well.[31] This study did not look at HD, so we can't say whether obese people would have done better on that. The larger you are, the more treatment you need, so standard in-center HD is not likely to be enough. If you are overweight and have diabetes, PD seems to be a better choice if you are younger—not older. A review of large studies found that in the U.S., if you are older than 45 and have diabetes, you are likely to live longer on HD than PD. In other parts of the world, survival was the same for both treatments.[32]

■ **Have a Hernia** – A hernia is a weak spot in the muscle of your belly. On PD, a hernia can be a problem if pressure from fluid in your abdomen traps part of your peritoneum in the weak spot—or if PD fluid leaks into your groin. Can you do PD with a hernia? Yes—once it is fixed. Among 122 people who started CAPD from 1994 to 2001, 17.2% had a hernia (some had more than one). Nearly three fourths were found *before* PD was started.[33] Most were fixed under local anesthesia with mesh to repair the weak spot, and a PD catheter was put in at the same time. In a study of 46 people who had hernias fixed, just one had to change to HD. This study found that the mesh repair was safe and effective.[34]

If you get a hernia after you start PD, you don't *have* to change to HD while it is fixed. A study looked at hernia repairs on PD over 10 years. People had no dialysis for 48 hours after surgery. Then they did a form of PD called *low-volume, recumbent-only*, or LVRO (recumbent means laying flat).

- Those doing **CAPD** did PD 3 days a week for 2 weeks, using a cycler for 10 hours at night. The cycler did 10 1-liter exchanges each night. For 2 more weeks, they did five low volume (1-1.5 liter) exchanges by hand per day. Then they went back to their normal schedule.

- Those using a **cycler** did PD 3 days per week for *one* week using a cycler for 10 hours at night. For 4 more weeks, they used the cycler 3 nights per week. Then they went back to their normal schedule.

No one in the study had a leak or an early recurrence of a hernia.[35]

Lying flat while you do PD exchanges when you heal from a hernia repair can reduce the pressure on your stitches. It takes 6 weeks for new collagen to fully form so the repair is stable, so lying down for PD for 6 weeks may reduce the chance of your hernia coming back. And, of course, after a hernia is fixed, you will need to strictly follow any limits you are given on lifting, jumping, driving, straining to have a bowel movement, or any other task that would raise the pressure in your belly.

PD: Wendy's Story

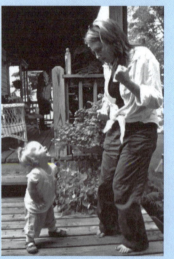

My name is Wendy. I am 39. I was diagnosed with Lupus at the age of 15, back in 1985.

I was a typical, difficult, "know-it-all" teen, and my doctors and my parents had a tough time getting through to me about just how serious my kidney problem was. It took years before I understood. In time, I adjusted, and was able to manage my lupus while my kidney problems stayed in the background. Around 2000, my kidney function began to drop faster. I was getting close to decision time.

In 2008, with my nephrologists, I began to research and think about types of dialysis. As a full time student looking forward to a career in mental health, I worried about being able to work and dialyze, not to mention being able to have a life outside my treatment.

After careful thought about the pros and cons of HD (in-center, nocturnal, home) and PD, I chose CCPD.

I had my catheter placed in February of 2009. I chose to have it placed above my beltline, on my left side. If I had it to do over again, I think I would have had it placed below my belt line. But, this would be for more aesthetic (and bikini-wearing ☺) reasons, than for medical reasons. My catheter (that I have named "Cathy") works just fine where it is. I choose not to use the catheter belts for PD patients. Instead, I often tuck my catheter into my underwear, and usually wear camisoles under my shirts.

I began (as many patients do) CAPD in March of 2009. After learning how to do manual exchanges, I switched to CCPD. Although I was very worried about the impact PD would have on me, I have found that it really has very little impact on my day-to-day life. I am so lucky to be able to benefit from CCPD. I feel *soooo* much better now than I did pre-dialysis. I never realized just how drained and unhealthy I was until I began to get rid of all those toxins!

A typical PD night looks like this:

- Every evening I place my bags of PD fluid on my CCPD cycler machine, turn it on, and set up "the deal" as I like to call it. This involves hooking up my bags to their respective tubing, and takes 5-10 minutes.

- I then go about my business (reading, cooking, watching some favorite shows) until I am ready to hook up for the night.

- Because I get up at 6 am, and my PD prescription (yours may differ) is 9 hours each night, I hook up at 9 pm. Then I turn on my machine and let it do the work. It will fill me with solution and drain it 3 times during the night. I don't need to do a thing. Because the tubing that connects me to the machines is about 12 feet long, I can go pretty much anywhere in my apartment (can't quite reach the fridge, though ☺).

- If I really want to, I can unhook from the machine until it is time for me to drain (about 1 hour and 40 minutes). So, despite what some people may think, I am not "chained" to my bed at all. Then, I can hook back up and go to sleep.

- I sleep on my side and my stomach. Rarely does the tubing ever get kinked. If it does, the machine sounds a little alarm. I shake the tube out and go back to sleep.

- In the morning, I wake up, unhook, and get ready for work. Easy peasy.

As far as supplies go, yes, there are many boxes. I have an entire closet in my home for my PD supplies. But, I have people over to my home on a regular basis, and most never have any idea I am on PD.

I am able to travel (cross country and soon overseas) quite easily on CCPD. My solution is sent wherever I go (in the U.S.) at no extra cost to me. I can also check my cycler as baggage at no extra cost (the airlines allow medical devices to be checked free of charge). This may be the biggest blessing of CCPD for me. I love to travel, and it is a big part of how I am able to feel "normal."

I am extraordinarily grateful to be able to use CCPD, and feel blessed at the technology and advances in medicine that allow me to keep living my life to the fullest.

Your Lifestyle on PD

We said in the intro of this book that your choice of a treatment option would affect every aspect of your lifestyle. In the case of PD, here's how:

Time Commitment

Each PD exchange done by hand takes about 30 minutes—and then your treatment goes on while you go about your day. All in all, your weekly time would look a lot like this:

Table 7-2: Time commitment for CAPD

Task	Time	Number of Exchanges/Week	Total
PD exchange	30 min	28	14 hours
Set-up/clean-up	10 min	28	4⅔ hours
Recovery time to feel well again	0	28	0 hours
			18–19 hours

Besides the **18 or 19 hours** per week you would need for PD exchanges, you'd also need time to order and receive supplies and wait for them to be delivered, go to your clinic to have blood tests done, and go back to meet with your care team.

If you use a cycler at night, the amount of time you are connected will depend on your prescription. In most cases, you can keep your connected time to 9 hours or less per night, or unhook after a fill and hook up again when you go to bed.

- **Exchange time for cycler PD**: 9 hours per night x 7 nights
- **Set-up/clean up**: 10 minutes x 7 nights = 1 hour and 10 minutes
- **Recovery time**: None
- **Total: 64 hours** and **10 minutes**

This seems longer, but all of the cycler time is at night while you're sleeping. You'd also need to set up and clean up the cycler, order supplies, wait for them, and fit in a clinic visit. You might have some daytime PD hours if you do a mid-day exchange by hand.

How You'll Feel During and After Treatment

When you first start PD and begin to put fluid in, you may feel very full—even stretched. Most people get used to this in a week or two. Lying down while you do exchanges can reduce the feeling of pressure while you adjust. You can also ask your PD training nurse if you can start with smaller bags of fluid and then go to larger ones if this is a problem for you.

Most people don't notice big changes in their energy or how they feel from hour-to-hour or day-to-day on PD. Since treatment is going on most or all of the time, it is very gentle.

Eating and Drinking

PD is continuous (CAPD) or done every night (CCPD or APD). This means your food choices and fluid intake can be much more liberal than with standard HD. Some people on PD have *no* limits and can eat and drink a normal diet. Others find that if they eat too much salt they retain fluid or get thirsty and drink too much. Or, if they eat too many foods with phosphorus, they start to itch. Your blood test results will guide what the dietitian tells you about what you can safely eat and drink.

Sugar in PD dialysate can give you a few hundred extra calories each day. Some people on PD struggle with weight gain. You can help prevent this by staying active and eating fewer starchy carbs like sweets, baked goods, rice, corn, or potatoes. PD fluid comes in three strengths:

- **1.5% glucose (sugar)**
- **2.5% glucose**
- **4.25% glucose**

The higher strength removes more water because it has more sugar. The 4.25% fluid gives you many more calories, *and* it is harder on your peritoneum over time. It's best to manage your PD so you can use the weakest strength of fluid as often as possible. (See Weight Gain, on page 102.)

Having your belly full of fluid can reduce your appetite—but it is vital to eat enough protein to keep your serum albumin level at or above 4.0 g/dL, or you may risk malnutrition. Since PD is the only type of dialysis that removes protein-bound wastes, you lose a little protein with each exchange. A dietitian can help you think of protein snacks or suggest other tips or products to help you get enough protein.

Medications

Most people who do standard in-center HD in the U.S. must take (and pay for) an average of 8 to 12 different prescription drugs each day.[36] While we could not find a study on use of drugs in people on PD from the U.S., a study from China found an average of just 3 to 6 different drugs[37]—about half as many—in 266 people on PD.

A large number of the drugs taken by people on HD are for blood pressure control. As a continuous, gentle treatment, PD itself can control blood pressure well, especially if icodextrin fluid is used and there is not a long daytime dwell with sugar-based fluid.[38] This can mean taking fewer (or no) blood pressure pills on PD.

Phosphate binders also make up a large number of the drugs taken by people on HD. People on PD may tend to have lower levels of phosphate[39]—which can mean fewer binders to take as well. These are some of the types of drugs that are common for people on PD:

- **Cholesterol medications** – to help prevent damage to your heart.
- **Cinacalcet (Sensipar®)** – to help treat too-high levels of parathyroid hormone that can cause bone disease.
- **Erythropoiesis stimulating agents (ESAs)** – injections to treat anemia (a shortage of red blood cells) by making more red blood cells. Treating anemia can give you more energy.

- **Iron** – to provide the building blocks to make red blood cells.
- **Phosphate binders** – antacids or special drugs taken to help your body get rid of extra phosphorus that can cause itching and long-term bone problems. People on PD may not need as many binders as those on standard HD.
- **Renal vitamins** – with kidney failure, "normal" vitamins could build up to toxic levels.
- **Vitamin D** – to help your body use calcium better and help avoid bone problems.

If you have diabetes, the sugar in the PD fluid is likely to affect your need for medications. Talk to a diabetes educator or doctor about what types of changes to make and what to watch out for.

Working

How old are you? Each year, half of all people in the U.S. who start dialysis are under 65, or "working age." As we've learned, nearly 92% of U.S. dialysis is done as standard in-center HD. Fewer than 1 in 4 working age people who do standard in-center HD are able to keep a job after they start treatment.[40] For many, this means taking Social Security Disability (SSDI), which pays only about 35% of what they earned at work. (The more you earn, the less SSDI replaces.) Job loss can push a family into poverty.

PD, on the other hand, is what we call a "work-friendly" treatment option. You can do an exchange at work in a clean office or use a cycler at night, so your days are free for work. Some people don't even tell their employers that they are on dialysis. There is no rule that says you must. People have done PD exchanges in cars and hotels. Supplies can be shipped ahead, making work travel fairly easy.

With your energy levels constant on PD, you won't have the ups and downs of standard in-center HD, which make some people feel like they can't get much work done. Among more than 163,000 working-age people with kidney failure, people who kept their jobs were much more likely to have chosen PD or had a transplant than to be doing standard in-center HD.[41]

Keeping a job may also mean keeping an employer group health plan (EGHP). An EGHP will pay first for the first 30 months that you are eligible for Medicare, whether you take Medicare or not. Medicare pays second during this time. Having both means fewer out-of-pocket costs for you, and more income to pay them with.

You may be able to use vacation or sick days to have a PD catheter placed, recover, and train for PD. If you know this is coming, you can plan to save up days. Or, if your company has 50 or more employees, you may be able to use the Family and Medical Leave Act (FMLA) to ask for unpaid time off. Plan on one clinic visit per month to do blood tests, and one more to check your blood pressure, review your treatment logs, and see if any changes are needed. Someone will also have to plan to be home one half-day per month for supply delivery. It may be possible to schedule your clinic visit and supply drop on the same day, to miss less work.

Doing your treatments just as you're taught will help you avoid infection—which could make you miss work.

Travel

When you do your own treatment, and it's portable, you can travel without having to plan months in advance. Toss your supplies in the trunk of your car, or call your supply company ahead of time to ship them to your destination. Shipping in the continental U.S. is free. Shipping to Hawaii, Alaska, or other countries may cost you money—but since the companies that make PD supplies work all over the world, you can go nearly anywhere.

There *are* challenges. Boxes of PD fluid are heavy. Hotels may charge a fee to receive your boxes. And, you still have to make time for your exchanges—even on vacation. But PD tends to take less time out of your life than standard in-center HD, and makes it easier to travel.

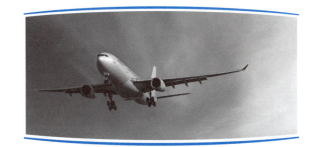

Most PD cyclers weigh about 30 or 40 lbs. and come with a carrying case. A small cycler can fit under an airplane seat or in an overhead bin. Or, you can check it as luggage. The Air Carrier Access Act (ACAA) of 1990 says *airlines can't discriminate against people with disabilities*. The law applies to U.S. and foreign flights.

The U.S. Dept. of Transportation (DOT) oversees air travel and has rules under the ACAA to help people with disabilities travel by air. These rules, called **14 CFR Part 382**[42] cover your rights when you need an "**Assistive Device**"[43]—like a portable dialysis machine.

Your rights include:

- **Not counting your machine as a carry on item** if it fits in the overhead bin or under the seat in front of you on the plane (Section 382.41(d)).
- **Help to stow and retrieve your machine as a carry on** (382.39(b5)).
- **Stowing your machine so it is one of the first things off the plane at the end of the flight**, if you checked it as luggage (382.41(f2)).
- **Giving your machine priority over other bags** if space is limited (382.41(f3)).
- **Baggage liability limits don't apply if the airline loses or harms your machine**—they must pay for your machine based on the purchase price (382.43(b)).
- **You can't be asked to sign a waiver of liability for loss or damage** (382.43c)).

Your rights when you check a cycler as luggage are less well known. Some agents will try to charge a fee if you have suitcases plus a machine (NOTE: With fuel prices high, most airlines now charge a fee for checked bags). Some will charge you if your machine weighs more than 50 lbs. Some do both.

DOT spokesman Bill Mosley says, "*We've told carriers that they shouldn't charge for dialysis machines, which are assistive devices*." **Under the ACAA (Section 382.57), the airlines are not allowed to charge you for your dialysis machine.**[44] Here is the section of the manual that tells the airlines that they can't charge you:[45]

Question: Are airlines allowed to charge for providing services to passengers with disabilities?

Answer: Airlines are not allowed to charge passengers for providing services or accommodations required by part 382, but may charge for optional services or accommodations. Examples of required services for which carriers may *not* charge are assistance with enplaning, deplaning, and making flight connections, and the *carriage of assistive devices* (including the provision of hazardous materials packaging for wheelchair batteries, when appropriate). Examples of optional services for which carriers may charge are the provision of in-flight medical oxygen and stretcher service. [Sec.382.57]

Preboard the Plane

As an assistive device, a PD cycler has priority for stowage. Measure it first so you know it will fit in an overhead bin or under the seat. If you plan to bring your cycler onto the plane, tell the gate agent, and ask for help to get your cycler on board and stowed if you need it. Gate checking may work IF the airline will give you the cycler back plane-side at your destination instead of having to pick it up at the baggage carousel. When boarding starts, the agent will ask for "*passengers who need extra time or assistance getting down the jetway.*" Board then, to be sure to have room to stow your machine.

About That Dialysate…

When you do PD, you'll need to bring dialysate on your trip, too. Plan ahead so your supply company can ship most of the boxes to where you will be staying. The airlines should take enough bags for a day or two of PD without a fee for extra or overweight luggage, but more than that will cost you money. All supplies must be in their original boxes, with the contents clearly labeled.

If you'll be staying in a hotel, call ahead and talk to the bell captain or hotel manager. Explain that you will need to receive life-saving medical supplies for your stay. Ask if they will waive the fee for accepting or storing packages (or charge you one fee, rather than per-box). Many hotels can provide a bathroom scale. It won't be as accurate as yours, but beats bringing one along.

If you do PD, you'll need to warm the bags so you don't get chilled by cold PD fluid. An electric heating pad won't take up much room in your suitcase. Lay a towel down above and below the heating pad and put the bag on top to warm it. Use the "low" setting.

Backup Care

You don't need to arrange for dialysis when you travel on PD, but it's a good idea to set up a back-up clinic that uses the supplies you are used to in case you run into a snag. Talk with your home training nurse or social worker to find one. It's also wise to do some homework about nearby hospitals and bring a copy of your medical records and meds list with you. Bring your emergency kit in case you get peritonitis.

Travel Tipping: When you travel with suitcases, the rule of thumb for tips is $1-2 per bag. When an item is heavy or you have many boxes, look for a Skycap with a large cart. He'll watch for your items, take them off of the baggage claim belt, load them onto the cart, and even help you find a cab. Plan to tip $5 for your machine plus $1 per box. You'll also have to tip the cab driver and the hotel bellman.

We hope your travel goes smoothly. But if you have a problem, you can report it to the DOT Disability Hotline at 1-800-778-4838 (voice) or 1-800-455-9880 (TTY).

Exercise

When you get extra sugar calories each day, exercise may help keep you from gaining weight. A study of more than 2,000 people on dialysis in the U.S. found that those on PD had fewer limits on what they could do physically than those who did standard in-center HD.[46] Exercise helps raise energy levels and can reduce depression. In one study, a 12-week walking program was started for people on PD. Compared to those in the control group, the walkers were less depressed.[47]

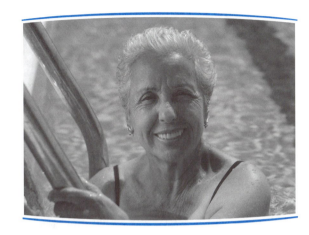

If your PD catheter is in your belly, you'll want to avoid raising the pressure in your abdomen—or drain and exercise while you're "dry." This can reduce your chance of getting a hernia. Upright cycling and weight lifting may be best done dry. If you like tennis, basketball, or other active sports, you may also find that you feel best dry—or the fluid would bounce around. Walking, bowling, dancing, Tai Chi…talk to your doctor first about your plans, but PD should not stop you from taking part in things you enjoy.

Swimming is a special case. Most clinics will ask you to swim only in an ocean or a private, chlorinated pool. Lakes, ponds, swimming holes, rivers, or public pools have more germs. Even in the ocean or a private pool, it's wise to put a waterproof Tegaderm® dressing or ostomy bag over your PD catheter. Once out of the water, wash up as you're taught, dry off, and use an antibiotic cream if your clinic suggests it. These steps will help keep you from getting an infection in your catheter or exit site.

Body Image

Any treatment for kidney failure—from PD to transplant—will require surgery, and will leave some new scars. With PD, there is no question that looking down and seeing a tube coming out of your body takes some getting used to. How you feel about yourself and about your body can affect your sexuality and how you relate to a partner.

If you have a partner, talk about your feelings. You may find that your loved one is so happy to have you around and able to do PD that the tube bothers *you* more than it does him or her. Some people cover the tube with gauze or a soft cotton belt so they don't have to look at it much. That's okay, too. Most people on PD do find that they get used to the catheter in time. Visit the *Sexuality and Fertility* module of **Kidney School**™ at www.kidneyschool.org to learn more about how to cope with a PD catheter.

Intimacy

Kidney failure affects hormone levels, and that includes sex hormone levels. As we said in Chapter 3, the more a treatment mimics healthy kidneys, the better you'll feel. Keep normal aging in mind, as well as other health concerns that can affect sexual function. Both of the leading causes of kidney failure—type 2 diabetes and high blood pressure—can cause sexual problems, especially in men.

Using a PD cycler at night does not have to stop you from being intimate. Of course you want to keep the tubing from getting kinked. And you might want to try out positions that don't put pressure on a full belly (spooning, or being side to side, for instance). There is also no rule that lovemaking must always occur at night, in a bedroom, or even in a bed at all.

With the 15% kidney function that PD provides, people who do PD have some sexual problems—but fewer than those who do standard in-center HD.[48]

For Women
One study in women found that 50% of healthy women and those with kidney transplants had some type of sexual dysfunction (problems with desire, arousal, or orgasm). On PD, the rate was 66.7%, while on standard in-center HD, it was 75%.[49]

For Men
Men on PD are more likely to have erectile dysfunction than healthy men.[50] In one study, *only* men on PD (not standard in-center HD) were able to get an erection when they took sildenafil (Viagra®).[51] In another, only two-thirds of men on standard in-center HD responded to sildenafil—while 9 out of 11 on PD did.[52]

Fertility
If you don't want a baby and you are of child bearing (or fathering) age, you'll need to use birth control when you're sexually active. Pregnancy is less likely on PD, but it can happen.

If you do want a baby, being a woman on PD can make pregnancy less likely. Any pregnancy in a woman on dialysis is considered high risk. In women, fibrous thickening of the surface of the ovaries has been found.[53] This may make it harder to release an egg. Some doctors think that having PD fluid in your belly could wash away an egg when you ovulate, which can make it harder to get pregnant. Small numbers of women *have* become pregnant on PD and delivered healthy babies.[54, 55] A study from Taiwan of 131 pregnancies among women on dialysis found about the same rates of success with PD (64.2%) as with standard in-center HD (70.9%).[56]

Sleep
PD and standard in-center HD have about the same level of sleep problems.[57] In a study of 124 people on PD, 43.5% said they had poor sleep quality—and those who did were more prone to depression.[58] If you are on PD and have *sleep apnea* (a condition where you stop breathing many times each night), using a PD cycler may help. A study done in a sleep lab compared people doing CAPD and CCPD. CCPD removed much more water from the blood. Only 4.2% of people on CCPD had sleep apnea vs. 33.3% on CAPD.[59]

It can take time to get used to sleeping with a PD cycler going. The cycler can wake you up with alarms, or the feeling of the fluid flowing in and out. Some people feel a pinch at the end of a drain cycle that can wake them up. You may even need to get used to a new sleep position if you slept on your stomach before and no longer can. Using a PD belt can help make the catheter more comfortable at night when you sleep. In time, you may reach the point where the cycler's swooshing noises *help* you fall asleep. A cycler should not squeak or squeal—if yours does, it may need repair or replacement.

Benefits of PD

Preserve Kidney Function Longer with PD

In most cases, kidneys don't lose 100% of their function when they fail—at least not right away. Having some natural kidney function can help you to feel better[60] and live longer.[61, 62] In fact, one study found that each 1% of kidney function you keep cuts your risk of death in half.[60] PD may help you keep your remaining kidney function longer than standard in-center HD.[63-65] It is vital to do PD just as you are taught and avoid *peritonitis* infection, though. Peritonitis can cause a *faster* loss of kidney function.[66] Residual kidney function does tend to drop over time. If you choose PD, your residual kidney function should be checked with a 24 hour urine test quite often until you don't make urine any more. Your PD dose will need to go up as your kidney function drops.

PD May Improve Your Chance of Transplant

If you plan to get a kidney transplant, PD may be good news for you. A study of more than 252,000 adult U.S. dialysis and transplant patients found that people on PD were about 40% more likely to get a transplant than those on standard in-center HD. This was true even after the researchers adjusted for differences between patients on standard in-center HD vs. PD.[41]

PD is an excellent "bridge" to transplant, because you do the treatments yourself. With a transplant, you will need to take a number of drugs. Doing PD shows the transplant team that you will care for a transplant well. Also, working age people on PD are more likely to have a job that may carry health insurance. Having a health plan helps pay for costly transplant drugs along with Medicare, or after Medicare stops (36 months after a transplant if kidney disease was the only reason you had it).

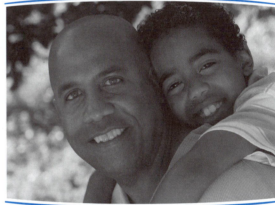

Medicare Starts Sooner with PD

There is another plus of PD—or any form of home dialysis. *You can get Medicare to cover your treatments from day one if you start home training before your 3rd full month of dialysis.** With standard in-center HD, Medicare will not kick in until the first day of your 3rd month of treatment. The dialysis bills can add up to tens of thousands of dollars for you in those first 3 months, especially if you don't have other insurance.

*You need to qualify for Medicare by working enough quarters, based on your age.

PD Makes Parenting Easier

If you have very young or even school-aged children, there will be days when a standard in-center HD schedule will simply not fit your life. A child can become ill in the middle of the night and need to stay home from school or daycare. There may be a play, band concert, or sports event that you would have to miss because it's on a treatment day. It can be hard—and costly—to find child care for school days off, vacations, and summer break.

The beauty of PD is that it is flexible to fit your needs. You can shift your exchange times a bit if you need to, so you can go to special events with your child. If you use a cycler at night, an extra-long tubing set will let you reach your child if he or she has a bad dream or a tummy ache. Children can and do get used to a parent doing dialysis—it just becomes another part of life.

PD Buys You Time

Even if you choose PD, a day may come when you must switch to HD. Choosing PD first can allow you time to get a fistula placed and have it ready to go, just in case. This means you may be able to avoid a hemodialysis catheter—with its very high risk of infection and death.

Problems or Complications of PD

It would be great if everything went smoothly all the time. But, some people who choose PD get off to a rough start. A catheter is placed but it won't drain and needs to be moved—another surgery. Or the catheter rubs inside the abdomen, which is uncomfortable. Infection of the catheter tunnel can occur when the catheter is put in. If you read about HD access, you know that problems can occur there, too. These problems can be solved.

Catheter migration

Sometimes a PD catheter won't stay down in the abdomen where it belongs. It may drift up under your ribs, where it can cause pain and may drain poorly. An X-ray will show this. The catheter may move back down by itself. This is often the case if you are constipated and take a laxative. Rarely, surgery is needed to move the catheter back where it belongs.

Problems draining

In rare cases, blood clots, fibrin, and/or omentum tissue can block the catheter so it won't drain. The omentum is a fold of the peritoneum that forms an apron of loose tissue. If omentum is in the way, a surgeon can trim or remove it using a laparoscope (Band-aid surgery). Enzyme drugs or heparin may be able to break up clots or fibrin.

Hernia

The extra pressure of fluid in the belly can cause or reveal a *hernia*—a weak spot in the muscle of the abdomen or groin. There are four main types of hernia:[67]

1. **Inguinal** – groin
2. **Exit site** – where the catheter comes out of your body
3. **Umbilical** – belly button
4. **Other incision** – any other spot where you have had surgery on your abdomen

When you do PD, umbilical and inguinal hernias are the most common types. You can often see the bulge of a hernia. An umbilical hernia looks as if an "innie" belly button has become an "outie." Call your doctor if you see any new bumps or bulges in your belly. An inguinal hernia will bulge down into the groin, where you can feel it, but may not be able to see it. Having a hernia can cause pain while lifting, or a dull ache.

On PD, two hernia problems can become serious:

1. **A loop of bowel is caught** – A hernia is "strangulated" when part of the bowel slips through the hole and is trapped. If the blood supply is cut off to the bowel, gangrene can occur. This is a life-threatening emergency—and a good reason to have a hernia fixed sooner rather than later.

2. **PD fluid leaks out** – Having PD fluid in your belly raises the pressure in your abdomen. With a hernia, PD fluid may leak at the catheter exit site. Or, in men, an inguinal hernia that leaks due to the pressure of PD fluid in the belly can lead to painful swelling of the scrotum. Special X-ray imaging can help find this problem.

Peritonitis

Infection is a risk with each PD exchange, since there is an opening into the body. Many people are scared away from PD by infection horror stories, often told by HD staff. *Sepsis* (blood poisoning) occurs when germs get into the bloodstream and travel through your body. Sepsis can land you in the hospital for IV antibiotics—and it can be fatal.

The data show that you may be safer from sepsis with PD than with an HD catheter or graft:[4]

Table 7-3: Risk of Sepsis from Access

If you have this type of access:	You might be at risk for sepsis:
HD catheter	About every 6 months
HD graft	About every 18 months
HD fistula	About every 24 months
PD catheter	About every 24 months

With a PD catheter, as with an HD fistula, you may only be at risk for sepsis about once every 2 years. As with ALL statistics, the ones in Table 7-3 apply to *groups*—not to individuals. We know many people who have done PD and *never* had peritonitis (let alone sepsis).

Peritonitis is often painful—which is a blessing and a curse. No one wants pain, but pain or a fever and/or cloudy drain bag are signs that you have a problem. You can add antibiotics to your next bag of PD fluid, to treat the problem. Your clinic may give you meds to have on hand and put in your PD bag just in case. If not, call your PD nurse or doctor to get a prescription if you suspect a problem. Peritonitis can almost always be prevented by doing all of your PD exchange steps just as you are taught. The best PD programs only see peritonitis about once every 7 *patient years*. You can ask about your clinic's peritonitis rate.

Can you still do PD after a bout of peritonitis? Maybe. A severe infection can scar your membrane too much to do PD. This is a reason to catch it as early as you can. A recent study looked at people who had peritonitis in their first 3 months of PD vs. a group who did not. The early peritonitis group was almost twice as likely to die or to have to switch to HD as the others.[68] This suggests that good training and technique are key to PD success. Remember, both you *and* your PD nurse need to be confident that you can do all of the exchange steps the right way to avoid infection.

Encapsulating Peritoneal Sclerosis (EPS)

EPS is a rare condition in which a "web" of adhesions and scar tissue form. In a study of 111 people who had EPS, all but 12 had had peritonitis at least once. About half of them died.[69] Early detection and treatment can help improve outcomes in people with EPS—since the main risks are sepsis and bowel obstruction. One study used laparoscopy to check for EPS early. The three patients in the study were treated and did very well.[70] EPS really is rare: in a study of 7,618 people on PD, just 33 had it.[71] The risk of EPS is higher in people who have done PD for 8-10 years or more, and in those who have had frequent bouts of peritonitis.[72]

Treatment for EPS includes the drug tamoxifen, certain anti-rejection medications, and steroids to reduce inflammation. Surgery is needed if the bowel is blocked. A very old surgical technique called *Noble plication*, which involves neatly lining up the loops of the small bowel and stitching them in place, seems to help keep EPS from coming back.[72]

Weight Gain

Most PD solution uses dextrose—sugar, or glucose—to form the gradient you need to remove fluid. Sugar has calories. The higher strength PD fluid you use, the more calories you take in.

Table 7-4: Calories from PD Fluid[73]

Solution	Grams of Dextrose	Grams of Dextrose Absorbed	Calories per Exchange
1.5%	15	15 x 75% = 11.25	11.25 x 3.4 kcal/g = 38.25
2.5%	25	25 x 75% = 18.75	18.75 x 3.4 kcal/g = 63.75
4.25%	42.5	42.5 x 75% = 31.875	42.5 x 3.4 kcal/g = 144.5

If you use two 1.5% bags, one 2.5% bag, and one 4.25% bag in a day, you'd absorb about 285 extra calories. It takes an extra 3,500 calories to gain a pound, so you could gain a pound or two or three each *month* if you're not careful. Exercising and eating fewer starchy carbs—potatoes, rice, corn, bread, cookies, bagels, cake—can help you keep off extra weight. Ask your dietitian about baking with almond flour instead of wheat flour. With some care to watch portions (if you need to track your potassium or phosphorus intake), you can have buttery, delicious cookies or cakes with higher protein and fewer carbs. Watching your salt and fluid intake so you can use mostly 1.5% bags will help a lot, too.

Membrane Failure

You may recall from Chapter 5 that *advanced glycation endproducts* or AGEs can damage the peritoneum. In time, this aging can cause the membrane to fail—it is no longer able to filter out water and wastes. In Australia, PET scans are done every 6 months to detect this problem early. This is not the practice in the U.S. If your peritoneum starts to fail, it's time to plan ahead for your next treatment option. It's best to do this before you have no choice in the matter.

Cycler Issues

Some PD concerns are only found in people who use cyclers. If air gets into the PD tubing and into the body, it can cause a sharp pain in the shoulder. Air can also get into your abdomen when the PD catheter is placed. Your body will absorb the air in about a week. If you don't want to wait that long, call your PD nurse. You may be able to lie with your feet higher than your head (called Trendelenburg position) and drain out some of the air.

Drain pain can also be a challenge on a cycler. At the end of a drain, some people feel a painful pulling sensation that can awaken them from sleep. Using a "tidal" setting, where some fluid is left in, may help.

Survival with PD

In Chapter 5, we showed you a table of life expectancy with standard HD and PD. They were pretty much the same. Let's look at survival a little more closely. Table 7-5 shows the rate of first, second, and third year survival for standard HD and PD. Note that this is for all ages. Younger people can expect to live longer than older ones.[4]

Table 7-5: PD Survival

Year on Dialysis	Survival on Standard In-center HD	Survival on PD
1	79.6%	91%
2	65.9%	79.3%
3	54%	67%
5	34.9%	46.7%
10	10.5%	14.3%

It would seem that people who do PD live longer. In fact, though, we can't be sure. The small number of people who were even given the option of PD in the first place may have differed from those who did standard in-center HD. They may have been younger or been in better health when they started treatment.

In general, studies find that standard in-center HD and PD have about the same survival. People who have a body mass index (BMI) greater than 26 (overweight), may not do as well on PD over time.[74] PD does a much better job of fluid removal than standard in-center HD—but neither option removes as many wastes as longer or more frequent HD. Survival is the same for both manual and cycler PD.[75]

A few years ago, a study found that the risk of death was higher after the second year of PD than for standard in-center HD.[76] It helps to know some background about this study. One reason PD works is because it can help you keep the little bit of kidney function you may still have. PD may rely, in part, on still having some kidney function. This remaining function tends to drop over time—which can mean not getting enough PD unless the prescription is increased. The data for this study came from the years before national guidelines taught nephrologists to measure remaining kidney function. *Today, your kidney function should be checked three times in the first 6 months of PD.* Ask your doctor to be sure this happens. Your PD prescription can then be tweaked, if need be, to be sure you get at least the amount of PD that the guidelines suggest.

Wrapping Up PD

We know of people who have done PD for 10, 15, or even 20 years! Most people who choose PD get a transplant or change to some form of HD much sooner than that, though. Among 277 people on CAPD followed for 23 years, just 6% were still doing CAPD after about 7 and a half years. None of them had high BMI's.[77] Keep in mind that a treatment choice does not have to be permanent. It's a great idea to start on PD and buy time to get a transplant or an access for HD—or do PD for years if you like it and it suits your lifestyle.

Short Daily Home Hemodialysis

"For me, it's a simple matter of life vs. death. Everything else is icing on the cake."

—Rich Berkowitz, on short daily home HD

Short daily HD is the newest and fastest growing type of home dialysis in the U.S. Between 2004 and 2010, there has been 2,080% growth in the number of clinics that offer short daily home HD.[1] Why? Because people who get more treatment look and feel better. They tell others. Their *doctors* tell others. Largely by word of mouth, this treatment has been quickly spreading across the country. By the way, you do not have to buy the dialysis machine. ***When you do any type of home treatment, PD or HD, the clinic provides the machine***, ***supplies, and training***.

For short daily HD, you do 5–6 treatments per week, each 2.5–4 hours long—and, as always with dialysis, we believe longer is better. Since you do your treatments yourself at home (very few U.S. clinics offer this option in-center), you decide which days of the week and what time to do the treatments, as long as you fit them all in. You can arrange them to suit your life, instead of living your life around a schedule set by a clinic. So, you can do your treatment in the mornings some days, and in the evenings on other days. A dialysis clinic nurse trains you and offers 24/7 phone support. Once a month, you visit the clinic to talk to your doctor, the training nurse, dietitian, and social worker.

The 5–6 day per week treatment schedule means no 2-day "killer gap" weekend (see Chapter 6) without dialysis. With fluid removed most days, you never gain as much water weight. So, you never have to take off as much fluid. Short daily HD home treatments are more gentle and comfortable, and pose much less risk to your heart than standard in-center HD. Removal of small wastes, like urea, is better with 5–6 "first hours" of dialysis a week, when the gradient is greatest. Removal of large wastes (that take more time) is about the same as standard in-center HD. Like standard HD, short daily HD replaces about **15–17%** of kidney function—but in a way that feels much more like having healthy kidneys.[2]

Perhaps because there *are* more first hours of treatment, a computer model found that short daily HD was **16.9% better than standard HD** at clearing urea from the blood.[3] Short daily HD was **15.5% better at clearing creatinine** and **2.5% better at clearing B2M** than standard in-center HD.

Is short daily HD harder on your access? It doesn't seem to be. A study looked at 2,160 patient months—400 of them on short daily HD—and the risk of having an access fail, clot, or need repair. The risk of an access problem was *less* on short daily HD (11–20%) than it was with standard in-center HD (21–24%).[4]

The U.S. National Institutes of Health (NIH) funded a year-long randomized, controlled study that compared standard HD with short daily HD done in a clinic. Now, the results of this **Frequent Hemodialysis Network** (FHN) study are out—and they *prove* that more HD is better. In this study, the 125 people who did short daily HD treatments (in-center, for this study) had smaller left ventricles (a good thing) and better physical function than the 120 who did standard in-center HD. Their blood pressure and phosphorus levels were lower, too. Here are the significant findings after 12 months of the study:[5]

Table 8-1: Frequent Hemodialysis Network Study Findings

	Standard HD	Short Daily HD
Predialysis phosphorus	Down 0.08±0.14	Down .64±0.14
Physical function	0.2±0.8 points higher	3.4±0.8 points higher
Weekly average systolic BP (top blood pressure number)	Down 0.9±1.6 points	Down 9.2±1.5 points
Left ventricular mass	2.6±3.2 grams smaller	16.4±2.9 grams smaller

How Short Daily Home HD Works
Find a short daily HD Clinic

To do short daily home HD, you first need to find a clinic that offers it. There are about 5,000 dialysis clinics in the U.S., and, as of this writing, nearly 800—about 1 in 6—offer short daily home HD.

When you have to go to a clinic three times a week for treatment, having it near your home is a big deal. But when you do treatments at home, after you are done with training you only need to go to the clinic once a month for clinic visits. So, a home clinic can be as far away as you are willing to drive once a month. We know of people who drive 200 to 300 miles each month to get to a clinic that offers the type of treatment they want.

Some parts of the U.S.—especially the East and West Coasts—are well supplied with home dialysis. Other parts, like the West or many rural areas, are not. If you live in a region with poor coverage, you may need to get creative:

- Try calling a clinic near you that offers PD or *standard* (3 times per week) home HD and see if they might expand their program to add short daily home HD. Be persistent—you may have to follow up for a while to convince the clinic of your interest.

- If you are not tied to where you live now, think about moving closer to a clinic that will let you do the treatment you prefer.

- Check around to see if others in your area also want home treatments. Approach your clinic or nephrologist as a group. Consumer demand has gotten new programs started in other places—why not yours?

- Contact a clinic farther away from your home to see if they can train you. For example, one nonprofit dialysis corporation, Northwest Kidney Centers in Seattle, trains and follows home patients as far away as Alaska. Once you are trained, your local clinic or doctor may be able to do your monthly checks. Some clinics want you to live close enough for their tech to maintain your machine. But, some machines can be shipped back to the company if there are problems. Ask if this can be done if you live far away.

- Contact dialysis companies to see if they may be starting a new program in your area. (See Chapter 14 for phone numbers.)
- Write a letter to the editor of your local paper about the benefits of home dialysis—and the trouble you are having finding it nearby. Drawing attention to the problem may help get a new program going.

Talk to Your Doctor

The second step you'll need to take to do short daily home HD is to talk to your doctor. Some nephrologists are well versed in all of the treatment options and will support you. Others have never seen a person on home HD, and don't believe that non-medical people could do it. They fear losing control over your treatments, since they can't see them done in a clinic. You may have a sales job to do. This book can help you with that.

Having a Care Partner

Nearly all short daily home HD programs will require you to have a care partner who will train with you. With *standard* in-center HD, which may be all that most doctors know, treatments often cause blood pressure to drop. It would be a challenge to deal with low blood pressure on your own. You might pass out or have severe, painful muscle cramps. So, it makes sense to require that someone else be on hand.

Short daily HD is not the same as standard HD. Blood flow rates tend to be somewhat slower. This means that if the lines disconnect or a needle pulls out, there is time to respond. And, with less fluid removed at any one treatment, the chance of a blood pressure drop is rare unless more than 1 kilo of water is removed per hour. We know of people who safely do their treatments by themselves. One program that we know of requires a "Life Alert®" type button for people who dialyze alone. If they have a problem, they can push the button, which is on a necklace, to alert a neighbor or 911. This service can cost as little as $15 per month.

How to Find a Short Daily HD Clinic

To help people find a home dialysis clinic, we built a unique list of every clinic in the U.S. that offers home training. You can see the database on our Home Dialysis Central website at: http://locater.homedialysis.org. You can use this list in two ways:

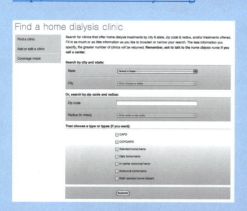

Find all the clinics in the U.S. that offer a treatment. You can do this by checking only the box for the treatment(s) you are looking for. So, to find out how many U.S. clinics do daily HD, check only that box, and click "Search."

Find all the clinics near you that offer a certain treatment. First, choose your state from the drop-down menu. Then, see if your city is in our list. If it is, select it or enter your zip code and check the boxes for the treatment(s) you are looking for.

If you don't get results—or if your city is not listed—re-do your search by state only. Leave the city blank and see what comes up.

If you do have a care partner, **it's best if *you* do as much as possible of your own treatments.** This is especially true of putting in the needles. Imagine how hard it would be for you to put needles into your care partner. You'd worry about hurting him or her, or causing an access problem. Home HD care partners tell us this is their *biggest stressor*. If you can't put in your own needles, tell your partner how much you value his or her help—and say it *often*. Your care partner can be an extra pair of hands or keep you company during some or all of the treatment. If he or she has to do all of the work, the chance for burnout is quite high—and you may need to find another treatment option. We'll talk about this more in Chapter 10.

Think about the timing of your treatments, too. If your partner needs to be on hand, even if he or she doesn't do *any* of the tasks, it takes time out of his or her day. Knowing *which* part of the day will be affected can make it easier to plan other events. Not planning ahead holds your partner's time hostage, which is not fair. So, talk about it.

In a recent study, we interviewed 13 people who did short daily home HD for at least 6 months, and then talked to their care partners.[6] We found four ways that couples were working together:

- **Couples who had strong relationships before short daily home HD grew even closer**. We called them *Thrivers*. They saw themselves as members of the same team, working to keep the person on dialysis healthy so they could both benefit. They spent quality time with each other during the treatments—playing cards, watching movies, or just catching up. (All of the people on dialysis in this group put in their own needles.)

- **Some couples struggled a bit to get started, but then did very well**. We called them *Survivors*. They called on their strengths to get through. One couple got counseling to help them communicate better, and said it helped a lot.

- **Some couples were not doing as well**. The care partner did most of the work, and felt put upon and burdened, "like a nurse" instead of a spouse. We called these care partners *Martyrs*. While this approach may work in the short term, it can lead to burnout in the long run.

- **One man was planning to go back to standard HD**. The husband, who was on short daily HD, was convinced that it was too hard on his wife—though she said it wasn't.

All of this tells us that good communication is key to successful short daily home HD—and successful relationships. If you and your care partner are doing well, doing short daily HD at home may help bring you even closer.

The Short Daily HD Machine

Most people who do short daily HD use a small machine that was built to be easy for home use. Right now, there is one machine on the market that was built for short daily HD in the home: the NxStage System One™. Most standard HD machines are about the size of a four drawer file cabinet and weigh 200–300 lbs. The NxStage System One is about the size of a microwave oven and weighs about 75 lbs. It has a handle, so with help to carry, it can be put in the trunk of a car so you can take it with you on trips.

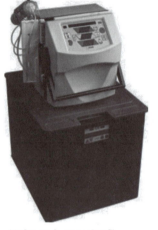

NxStage System One™
Photo courtesy of NxStage Medical, Inc.

If you have seen a standard HD machine, you know it looks complex. Just "stringing" the machine with the dialyzer and blood tubing can take time to learn. With the NxStage System One, the dialyzer and blood lines are built into a cartridge. You open the machine, drop the cartridge into place, and latch the machine closed. This makes a complex task simple. Because the NxStage machine was made to be easy to use, it takes less time to learn how to use it than a standard one.

You need dialysate for HD. The NxStage System One can use bags of sterile dialysate like PD. Or, the NxStage PureFlow™ SL makes enough high purity dialysate for 1–3 days of treatments, using your home tap water. The PureFlow was designed to use as an end-table, with the NxStage System One sitting on top of it. The NxStage System One uses a standard, grounded electrical outlet. The PureFlow can be plumbed into your home, or can use a standard faucet and outlet.

Other, standard machines can be used for short daily home HD, but since they take longer to set up and clean up, they may be too time consuming to use five or six times per week. Most standard HD machines also require complex water treatment systems, and special wiring and plumbing. Keep an eye out: a number of companies are working on small, portable home HD machines as we write this.

Setting Up a Treatment Room

We have seen people do short daily HD in tiny spare bedrooms, living rooms, pool decks, cruise ship cabins, sailboats, in RVs, and hotel rooms. In New Zealand and Australia, camper vans have been set up for dialysis and can be rented for holidays.

When you set up a space for short daily HD in your home, you'll want to figure out a way to sort out and store your supplies so you can get to them with the least amount of fuss. Some people use open bookcases or shelves. Some use dresser drawers; others use closed cupboards. Labels will help you keep track of what's where if you choose closed storage. In many programs, a home visit from the training nurse can help scope out which room might work well for you, and give you some tips about how to keep track of your supplies. We recommend a book written by a short daily HD care partner (Dr. Linda Gromko) and an interior designer (Jane McClure), called *Arranging Your Life when Dialysis Comes Home*. It's the only book we know of that helps people set up home dialysis treatment rooms. You can find it at: www.arrange2live.org.

Each month, you'll order and receive supplies. You'll learn how to keep track of what you have and figure out what you'll need. It's a good idea to keep some reserve supplies in case a storm, or other problem causes a delivery delay.

Short Daily Home HD Training

What to Expect

Learning to do home HD of any type is a *lot* like learning to drive a car. Driving was scary at first! There were things to do with your hands and your feet, buttons, lights, switches, and gauges. And, at the same time, you need to stay between the lines, follow the road signs, and avoid hitting anything. It's a lot to take in. For many of us, learning to drive took a few weeks and a driver's education class—plus lots of behind the wheel practice. After that, it may have taken months to really feel *confident* in our driving. But most of us are at a point now where we don't have to think about each step of driving a car—we just do it. Driving became a routine. It took some time, but we got there.

Like driver's education, training for short daily home HD may also take from 2–6 weeks. There is a lot to learn that's new to you. Learning to do HD can be overwhelming at first— *but it gets better in time.* One woman who is a care partner for her husband on short daily home HD suggested that while you are training, *clear your calendar* of optional events so you can focus. Make other things easy. Freeze food in advance, or get take-out if you can. Delay social gatherings. Put off your volunteer work for a while. You can pick all of those things back up again once you have found your new normal.

Training itself may be done with just you and a partner (or just you if the clinic permits this), or in small groups. We highly recommend small groups. They give you and your partner a built-in support group. Others may ask questions you didn't think of, and vice versa. And training a few people at a time can help reduce the long waits some clinics have for training slots. Plus, you *know* you're not alone when others train with you.

The training schedule is often during the work day. If you work, ask if the training program hours can be flexible or you and your care partner may need to rearrange your work hours or take a leave of absence. Part of the purpose of dialysis is to allow you to have a full life that includes work. Talk to your home training nurse if your job and health plan are at risk. Perhaps early morning, late afternoon, evening, or weekend times could be used for at least some of the training days. You'll do your treatments during the training sessions as well.

What You'll Learn

Most short daily home HD training programs focus on the nuts and bolts of how to do the treatment from start to finish. You'll learn to track and order supplies, and fill out treatment logs. And, you'll learn what to watch out for, what each alarm means, and what to do if you run into a snag. You'll get a lot of hands-on practice—and you won't go home until you, your partner, and your training nurse are all confident that you can do it. The training nurse may come to your home to watch your first treatment there, and you'll have someone to call 24/7 if you have questions.

This is a lot of information to take in, and there will be times when you don't think you can do it. *Nearly everyone who goes through the training feels this way at some point.* Most can push through it, gain the confidence they need, and succeed at home. If you have trouble, talk with your training nurse about your learning style and what works best for you. Having an overview of what you'll learn each day might help you see the big picture, for example. If you aren't sure why something is done, ask. You can learn a lot from mistakes, too! Don't be afraid to make some. Your training nurse will help you learn how to handle them.

Back-up Options

Standard in-center HD is always a back-up for short daily home HD. If your partner needs a break, has to go on a trip, or doesn't feel well, you can set up one or more treatments in the clinic. Depending on the clinic policy, you might even be able to bring your machine and do in-center self-care. If this is the case, you can help show others what short daily home HD is like and talk about how it makes you feel.

Supplies

The drivers who bring PD supplies will take them upstairs if need be and stack them where you want them. If you use a Fresenius machine for home HD, their drivers will put away your supplies, too. If you use the NxStage System One with bags, the driver will bring your supplies inside. If you use the PureFlow SL, your deliveries will be made by a parcel carrier. Your order will be brought to a first floor doorway, but if no one is home, it will be left in a safe place out of the weather.

Who Can Do Short Daily Home HD

There are only a few reasons why most people could not do some type of HD. As we said, in the U.S., standard in-center HD is the "default" treatment, though short daily home HD is far easier on your body and your heart. You need an access—fistula, graft, or catheter—to be able to do HD of any type. People who have dementia, cognitive impairments, use a ventilator, or are hard to transport may do *better* on short daily HD if a loved one is willing to be trained to give the treatments. Not having to go to a clinic three times each week can be a huge plus.

Short daily HD is nearly always done at home, because it is very hard to work out the logistics in a clinic. Most clinics will require the person on dialysis to have a partner. For this reason, most people who do short daily home HD are married, in a committed relationship, or have a family member, friend, or neighbor to help.

Others have gotten creative. If you have a spare room, you might trade free rent for HD help. Two people who do short daily HD could share a home and be each other's partners. Each would need his or her own machine and only one could do a treatment at a time. Those with the resources or a health or long-term care plan that will pay for it may hire a helper. (NOTE: Even if you hire a helper, it's still best for you to be the one who does the treatments if you are able.) Medicare does *not* pay for home HD helpers; other health or long-term care plans may.

We believe that anyone who is motivated can do short daily home HD. It might be a good choice for you if you:

- **Are caring for someone at home**
- **Have a job you want to keep**
- **Live far away from a clinic**
- **Are a student of any age**
- **Love to travel, or need to for work**
- **Need a flexible schedule for whatever reason**
- **Have a failed transplant**
- **Have complications of standard in-center HD: nerve damage, heart damage, blood pressure that is hard to control**
- **Are obese and can't get enough dialysis with standard in-center HD**
- **Want to have fewer diet and fluid limits**
- **Are pregnant—or you'd like to be**
- **Are a frail elderly person with a care partner who will help you**
- **Want control and are not happy with standard in-center HD**
- **Can no longer do PD**

Your health plan may be a reason that a clinic *won't* let you do short daily HD. If you have Medicare only with no secondary payer, or a health plan that refuses to pay for more than three treatments per week, you may have fewer options. Most clinics will offer short daily HD to anyone whom they believe will succeed with it, regardless of their insurance. Some won't. This is one of many reasons why it's best to keep a job with a health plan if you have one—it can give you more choices.

Stick to Your Guns

We have heard that some doctors or clinic staff will try to talk people out of doing home treatment. Some will even give bogus reasons why you "can't" do it. You might be told that you would have to get rid of your pets. Not true! Of course you can't do home HD if you are a hoarder or live in filth. You have to clean off your access well, wash your hands, and keep Fluffy from chewing or scratching your tubing or supplies. But we've seen people safely dialyze at home with a beloved pet asleep on their laps.

We've heard people say they can't do home HD because their homes aren't as clean as the clinic. Dialysis clinics *should* look clean—they are built with easy to wipe surfaces and are often white and shiny metal. But, like hospitals, clinics are hotbeds of germs. In most cases, you are *far less likely to get an infection at home than in a clinic.*

If you're reading this book for a loved one, who can't read, he or she may still be able to do home HD. Most people who can't read come up with ways to hide that fact from others. People have trained for home HD without their clinics even knowing that they couldn't read. Often, non-readers have come up with ways to help themselves learn. They may be very good at memorizing steps of a sequence, for example. The home training nurse can use pictures and lots of hands-on demonstrations to be sure that someone knows what needs to be done and can do it.

We truly hope that no one looks at you and decides you wouldn't be "suitable" for home HD because of your age, race, gender, tattoos or piercings, your sexual orientation, how much schooling you have, how much money you make, how you dress, or what color you dye your hair. None of these is a reason to deny you a treatment option that could help you feel better. If you believe that you are being discriminated against, talk to your doctor. Switch doctors if you need to. Contact your ESRD Network (we list them for you in Chapter 14). Don't give up!

Your Lifestyle on Short Daily Home HD

We said in the intro of this book that your choice of a treatment option would affect every aspect of your lifestyle. In the case of short daily HD, here's how:

Time Commitment

Most short daily HD treatments last 2.5–4 hours, plus set-up and clean-up time. All in all, your weekly hours would look like this:

Table 8-2: Time commitment for short daily HD

Task	Time	Number of Treatments	Total
HD treatment	2.5–4 hours	5–6	12.5–24 hours
Set-up/Clean-up	45 min	5–6	3.75–4.5 hours
Recovery time to feel well again	30 min	5–6	2.5–3 hours
			18.75–31.5 hours

Besides the 18.75–31.5 hours for treatments, set-up, and clean-up, you also need to count on some time once a month for a clinic visit, and to order, receive, and put away supplies. Short daily home HD adds up to a part-time job. But, since you can choose when to do the treatments, you can fit them into your life more easily than a fixed schedule set by a clinic.

How You'll Feel During and After Treatment

Like standard in-center HD, short daily home HD treatments should not hurt. If you have a fistula or a graft, you'll have needles. Most people who do short daily home HD and have a fistula use the Buttonhole technique to make placing the needles nearly painless (see page 50).

You are much less likely to feel cold on short daily home HD than standard in-center HD, because you don't need to have the dialysate as cold.

You are *far less* likely to have a blood pressure drop that could lead to cramps, vomiting, headaches, etc., since you remove less fluid at each treatment. This is why most people say they feel good just 30 minutes or so after a short daily HD treatment. You can get back a lot of quality time in your life by not losing the 6 or 7 hours of recovery after each standard in-center HD treatment. Keep in mind that if you start dialysis by going right to short daily home HD, it's going to feel as if you are losing time—not gaining it.

Eating and Drinking

Short daily HD removes fluid 5–6 days a week, so most people who do it have few or no fluid limits. Salt is less of an issue. Your food choices and fluid intake can be much more liberal than with standard in-center HD. Your blood test results will guide what the dietitian tells you about what you can safely eat and drink.

Short daily HD may or may not remove more phosphorus than standard HD or PD—studies have gone both ways on this.[7-9] So, you may still need binders, or you may need to limit foods that are high in phosphorus. In fact, since you'll likely have more energy and a better appetite, you might even need *more* binders.

Medications

Short daily HD is very good at managing fluid levels, which helps to protect your heart. Removing fluid nearly every day will help to control your blood pressure. Even during training, your doctor will probably start to cut back on your blood pressure pills. In time, most do not need them at all.[10]

These are some of the types of drugs that are common for people on short daily HD:

- **Cholesterol medications** – to help prevent damage to your heart.
- **Cinacalcet (Sensipar®)** – to help treat high levels of parathyroid hormone that can cause bone disease.
- **Erythropoeisis stimulating agents (ESAs)** – injections used to treat anemia (a shortage of red blood cells) by making more red blood cells. Treating anemia can give you more energy and help prevent heart damage.
- **Iron** – to provide the building blocks to make red blood cells.
- **Phosphate binders** – antacids or special drugs taken to help your body get rid of extra phosphorus that can cause itching and long-term bone problems.
- **Renal vitamins** – with kidney failure, "normal" vitamins could build up to toxic levels.
- **Vitamin D** – to help your body use calcium better and help avoid bone problems.

Working

We define a "work-friendly" treatment as one that lets you feel well enough to work and that doesn't interfere with your work day. Short daily home HD is a work-friendly treatment. People who do short daily home HD feel well and have more energy. And since treatments can be done before or after work, short daily HD fits into a standard work week without needing a lot of extra time off. Someone will need to be home one half-day per month to receive your supplies. We know of many people who were able to keep working or go back to work after they switched from standard in-center to short daily home HD.

Keeping you out of the hospital can also make a treatment work-friendly. A study was done of 42 people who switched from standard to short daily HD, for a total of 793 months of treatment over 6 years.[11] The group was chosen because they had a lot of illnesses to start with, and were not doing well on standard in-center HD. They had one-third fewer hospital days on short daily HD than before.

Miriam's Story: There's no Place Like Home

Miriam Lippel Blum

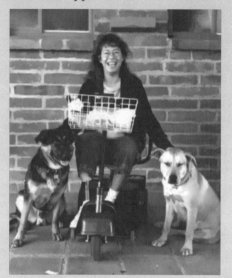

Adjusting to life on dialysis is never easy, no matter which choice—PD or HD—you make. For me, the benefits of home far outweigh the in-center model. Being in charge of treatments tailored to my needs gives me a sense of control, and the freedom, flexibility, and quality of life I did not have in-center.

I have been on dialysis since 1994. I spent 6 years on PD, 6 on in-center HD, and am now on short daily home HD. My kidneys failed when I was 34 after an allergic reaction to a medication caused interstitial nephritis. In a healthy person, this would have been the *start* of kidney damage. For me, with type 1 diabetes from the age of 10 with already damaged kidneys, it was the death knell of my kidney function.

When I was 28, my nephrologist said that some time in the future I might need dialysis. I knew very little about it, and decided to learn as much as I could, see what it was all about, and meet people who were doing it. I went to a medical library and read. Then I set up meetings at an in-center HD clinic and an outpatient PD clinic, speaking to patients on each treatment. There was no question in my mind after seeing all the options, that I would choose PD.

The people I met on PD seemed to have active lives: they worked, traveled, and looked much healthier than the standard HD folks. They were in charge of their own treatments and had more flexibility. I was a busy grad student in Los Angeles at the time, and couldn't imagine a life with the kind of limits standard HD would impose.

So, when my kidneys actually did fail 6 years later, I knew what I wanted. Luckily, there was no health reason to keep me from using PD, so I had a Tenchkoff catheter placed. The training was not hard. I learned quickly how to do the exchanges safely, add heparin and insulin into the fluid, give myself EPO, and take care of my catheter. I chose to do PD by hand four times a day. I was told it would be better for my cardiac status and didn't want to be attached to a machine for hours. I kept working and even did exchanges in my office on my lunch hour.

It took time to adjust to what my body felt and looked like with 2.5 liters of dialysate in my belly. I'm not a big person, so I looked pregnant, and it was hard when people asked me when the baby was due. I even had to buy slacks at a maternity store to find ones that would fit right. But I viewed it all as the price I had to pay for life, so my husband and I learned to live with the changes and challenges it brought.

Success with any home treatment really depends on attitude and willingness to take on your own care. Having knowledgeable and caring professionals to call upon helps, as does family support. But in the end, it's mostly up to you. I did what I had to, to take care of myself, but did not define my life by my disease. When not dealing with health issues, I lived as fully as I could. I worked 40+ hours per week at my job, sang in a choir, did aerobic dance three times a week, and my husband and I took trips to Maui, Utah, South Carolina, Arizona, and lots of places in California, too. It just took some careful planning. I shipped

PD fluid to hotels, packed all the meds and supplies, set up a back-up unit in case of problems, and brought health records, just in case.

After 6 years, I developed leaky hernias along an incision from a past surgery. My health at the time prevented surgical repair, and my only choice then was standard in-center HD. Home HD was not an option—it was not even offered then in Tucson, AZ, where my husband and I had moved. I had spent 5 years on the transplant list, with no match, then my cardiac status ruled out transplant as an option. So, to keep living, I had to get used to a life on standard in-center HD. This was extremely hard for me.

On a physical level, I never felt as well on standard in-center HD as I had on PD. The 2-to-3 day build-ups of toxins and fluids and 3-hour removal sessions were very taxing to my body. The treatment caused a great deal of inflammation in my blood vessels, causing major heart and circulation issues in short order. The diet and fluid limits were much stricter than PD, and I had to go back to multiple daily insulin injections.

The center's schedule was very rigid, restricting my life even more. Trying to change a time or date to celebrate holidays, or attend a concert—or for that matter any other social event—was always a huge hassle. But the worst thing for me was the time in the center itself. I never felt safe.

I was used to being in control of my own care, and found I was often more aware and careful than most of the techs in whose hands I was now entrusted. Depending on the luck of the draw, I could be faced with a competent tech or one who was not. I saw many errors. One night a tech almost injected me with 10 times the heparin dose that was prescribed. I caught the error at the last second and had to scream to get her to stop. Had I been a less educated patient, I would have likely died.

In my 6 years there, I saw many contamination and infection issues. There was understaffing that created rushed and stressed staff, and frequent turnover that created more and more less-experienced, poorly-trained or under-supervised techs.

Not a week went by when I didn't witness paramedics treating a fellow patient in crisis while in treatment. Sometimes the people returned and often, not. The tension wore on me and I dreaded being there.

I read a number of nephrology news magazines and websites and saw that home HD was becoming a choice. There was growing evidence that short daily HD seemed to have very good results. I started asking at my center if this would be an option there. They began to explore the issue, but it was clearly going to be a long time before they were ready. Meanwhile, I got on the waiting list for home HD training at a clinic in Scottsdale, AZ, about 2 hours from my home.

After a year, my husband and I started training at the DaVita clinic in Scottsdale. My husband, because of his work travel, can only be my care partner on the weekends. We were blessed to find a wonderful tech in Tucson who had just left in-center HD and was willing to work with us. We hired her and she trained with us. We were lucky to be able to pay for her help. Many can't afford this, and Medicare will not pay for a hired helper.

We moved to Scottsdale for 5 weeks to avoid the daily commute. It was costly, but we counted it as an investment in my life and health. The training was intense! My husband, our tech, and I learned all the ins and outs of how to safely run the NxStage System One™ machine; how to do buttonholes; to draw, process, and mail blood tests. We learned how to chart everything and deal with emergencies. The training nurses were tolerant, friendly, helpful—all one would expect from true professionals. We met other people doing home HD, too.

After 5 weeks, we were home with our machine to do it ourselves. The nurses are always on call by phone if there is a problem, as are NxStage staff. My husband helps me on Sundays and our technician does the weekdays. They set up the machine and help me connect to it. I put in my own needles and monitor the sessions.

Of course, there have been frustrations along the way. I had hoped that my sessions would be 2 to 3 hours long but need 4 hours to feel good, and that is how long I dialyze 6 days a week. The NxStage machine is "portable," but weighs a hefty 75 lbs. and is about the size of a 13-inch TV. That has limited travel for us. Another issue for me is the noise and the fact that every 30 minutes or so it goes through self-checks, when I must take and record blood pressure and vital signs. These interrupt my concentration and have made serious work hard for me to do.

We had hoped for some payment from our catastrophic care insurance for the costs of the tech, but were denied because we didn't use an agency to hire her. We are appealing. If you are thinking about doing home HD, some insurance companies will pay for a helper, so it is wise to check with them first and learn the rules.

I have made a life for myself on home HD. I am grateful to dialyze in a clean, quiet room in my home where I am not worried about exposure to others' infections and where the person who is helping me is a well-trained and competent partner.

Sometimes the simple comforts of life mean a great deal. I can have a friend over to spend time with while I dialyze, eat a light lunch, read, watch TV, listen to music, talk on the phone, nap, or work on my computer. I can shift the timing of my sessions to meet my needs. Most of all, I feel much better than when I was on standard in-center HD. Because I dialyze 6 days a week, I have less fluid to remove and fewer toxins in my body. There is less fluctuation of blood chemistry and I am not so exhausted.

I have had no hospitalizations since I have been at home. My skin color became less sallow and I heal faster. I have the energy to exercise at a gym 6 days a week and can keep up a full day's activity. I can enjoy my free time more because I feel so much better. The positive impact of home HD on my health is clear to all who know me.

Every dialysis nurse and tech I have ever spoken to about home HD or PD has said that if they had to be on dialysis, they would choose a self-care option, too. I think that speaks volumes!

Ms. Lippel Blum is a freelance writer and poet, based in Tucson, Arizona. She has been dialyzing at her home with the NxStage System One since 2006.

Travel

With short daily home HD, you can travel by car, air, or boat for long or short stays. (We're not sure about trains or buses, but it's worth checking.) As with PD, NxStage will ship bags of dialysate to your destination. This service is free if you travel in the continental U.S. For trips to Alaska or Hawaii, you will have to pay for shipping. For a long stay, you may want to think about shipping the PureFlow device instead of a pallet full of boxes of fluid bags—it weighs less, so shipping may be less costly. Talk to NxStage about which shipping companies may offer you the best deal. At this time, NxStage does not support travel outside of the U.S. Since the NxStage machine is now used in many other countries, the company may start to do so in the future.

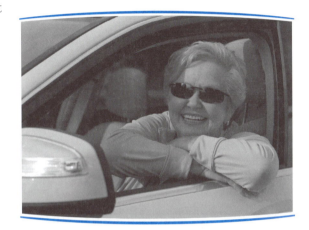

For short trips, you can load the NxStage System One into the trunk of a car with some bags of fluid and supplies, and hit the road. Bring your medical records along, and talk with your social worker about having a back-up clinic in case you forget something or run into a snag.

At about the size of a microwave oven, the NxStage machine is small enough to take along on a cruise. On an airplane, you can check it as "lifesaving medical supplies" at no charge (see page 95).

Another option for travel is to set up standard in-center HD. If you do this, be sure to talk with your dietitian—you may need to reduce the amount of potassium in your diet on your trip since you will only be getting treatment half as often.

Exercise

A small study of just 10 people who switched from standard in-center HD to short daily HD did not find a difference in their exercise endurance.[12]

Body Image

Body image concerns related to having a fistula, graft, or catheter for HD will be the same for short daily HD as for standard HD. We have been impressed to see that skin color often returns to a healthy pink with short daily HD, though, which can help boost your self-esteem and feelings of being normal.

Intimacy

Better fluid removal that controls blood pressure may help improve sexual function, especially in men. Both men and women may have more overall energy and more active lives—both in and outside the bedroom. Not many studies have yet been done on sexual function with short daily HD. A report from Italy found that both well-being and libido improved more than expected after people switched from standard to short daily HD. The results were good enough that the clinic chose to keep offering the option.[13]

If the cause of your kidney function can harm your blood vessels (like diabetes or high blood pressure), you may have damage that will persist even after doing short daily home HD. Spending a longer time on standard in-center HD may also make it hard for your body to benefit from a change.

Fertility

Your chances of fathering a child if you are a man, or of getting pregnant and having a healthy baby if you are a woman, are better with 20 hours or more of HD per week. As we noted in Chapter 4, there are a handful of case reports of women having healthy babies on short daily HD. [14-17]

Sleep

Short daily HD may help you sleep better. A study that followed 127 people found that after doing this treatment for a year, they:[18]

- Slept more soundly at night
- Were less sleepy during the day
- Had fewer symptoms of restless legs syndrome (RLS)

In this study, people did not sleep any longer. And, they needed just as many sleeping pills to help them sleep. But, overall, they did sleep better.

Benefits of Short Daily Home HD

As you may have guessed by reading this far, there are a number of benefits to doing HD more often. Some studies tested people on standard in-center HD, then followed them onto short daily HD. This before-and-after, or "pre-post," study design is a good way to see if the treatment switch makes a real difference. Here is what we learned:

Overall Well-being

Small studies have found better well-being with short daily home HD. One study followed 12 people from standard in-center HD (4 weeks) to short daily HD (8 weeks) and then back to standard HD (4 weeks). During short daily HD, more urea was removed. Eight of the 12 had symptoms during standard in-center HD that partly or fully vanished during short daily HD—and came back when they went back on standard in-center HD. Average blood pressure was much lower during short daily HD, too.[20] Another U.S. study followed 21 people who did 4 weeks of standard in-center HD and then 4 weeks of short daily HD. They found better blood pressure, fewer symptoms between treatments, and more urea removal. There were also fewer machine alarms. Nutrition and quality of life began to improve. This study did not find any increase in vascular access problems.[21] The NxStage FREEDOM study found much less depression among 128 people doing short daily home HD.[22]

Better Fluid Removal and Heart Health

Short daily HD is much better than standard HD at removing fluid. Among 11 people who did short daily HD for 18 months, blood pressure was much lower than it had been on standard HD. The study participants gained less fluid between treatments, and had less interstitial fluid—they got drier. As a result, they took 60% fewer blood pressure pills in the first month, and even fewer as time went on. And, their homocysteine levels— a marker of heart disease—were lower.[23]

To look at heart disease risk, researchers in Italy switched 12 people with high blood pressure who'd been on standard in-center HD for 6 months or more to short daily HD for 6 months. On short daily HD, they had much lower blood pressure and interstitial fluid. Most were able to stop taking their blood pressure pills.[10]

In the short run, better blood pressure control should mean less risk of a blood pressure drop during treatment, with fewer cramps, headaches, less vomiting, etc. And, it does. In a small study, 6 people who had severe blood pressure drops during treatment did standard in-center HD for 12 weeks, short daily HD for 12 weeks, and then standard in-center HD for 12 weeks. Five of the six had diabetes. On short daily HD, their blood pressure drops *disappeared*. People lost much more fluid weight and needed less saline during their treatments. They were able to stop taking blood pressure pills. When they went back on standard in-center HD, all of their symptoms came back—and 5 of the 6 had to go back on blood pressure pills.[24]

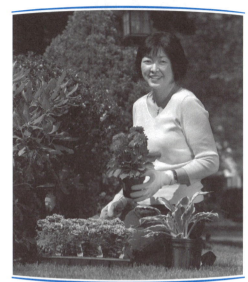

Better blood pressure control helps prevent—or reverse—damage to the heart's left main pumping chamber, called *left ventricular hypertrophy*, or LVH). So, with better blood pressure control, people who do short daily HD should have less LVH. And, they do. In a study of 26 people on short daily HD and 51 on standard in-center HD, both groups had similar heart tests at the start. After a year, those doing standard in-center HD were the same. But those doing short daily HD had left ventricles that were 30% smaller. Their phosphate levels were lower, and so were their C-reactive protein levels (a marker of heart disease).[25] Researchers in Canada followed people on short daily HD for up to 6 years. They found that all of the earlier benefits they'd found were still there—and that LVH was reversed.[26]

Waste Removal

Looking at just urea, short daily HD removes more than standard in-center HD.[27] Of course, we know that urea is not the only—or even the most important—waste that dialysis removes. A computer model of standard in-center HD vs. short daily HD found that short daily HD should remove more urea, creatinine, and B2M.[28] Does it? A study was done of 14 people on standard in-center HD for 6 months who then switched to short daily HD for 6 months. On short daily HD, urea and creatinine really were lower. Uric acid was also lower, and so were levels of some protein-bound wastes, including p-cresol.[29] Nocturnal HD does the best job of removing wastes.

Improved Nutrition and Appetite

How well you can eat says a lot about how you feel. In a study of 8 people who switched from standard in-center to short daily HD, their protein levels (*albumin*) rose. They gained a couple of kilos of "real" body weight, and had more lean body mass (muscle).[30] Their total cholesterol went up, too, perhaps because they were eating better. A study by the same group of researchers noted that people on short daily HD had an appetite for food again. This might have been because they felt better, had fewer diet limits, and did not need to take as many pills.[31] Another study of 17 people who switched from standard in-center to short daily HD also found higher protein levels, since they ate more protein. They also had an increase in real body weight.[32]

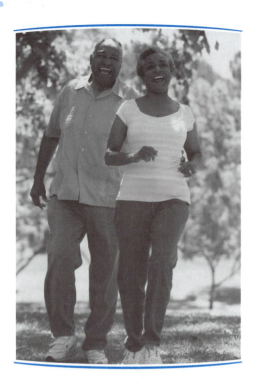

Better Quality of Life

What happens when you have better fluid and waste removal and your appetite is improved? When you have control over your schedule, more energy, and the chance to work toward your goals? You tend to have better health-related quality of life (HRQOL). HRQOL means that you say (by filling out a survey) that your physical and mental function are better, and you feel less burdened by kidney failure. On dialysis, when HRQOL is better, you will be less likely to be in the hospital and more likely to live longer.[33]

In a study that compared 11 people on short daily HD to 22 people on standard in-center HD, those on short daily HD had better HRQOL. They also had fewer symptoms—fewer blood pressure drops with cramping and headaches. They gained less fluid between treatments and had fewer fluid limits. They were less dizzy, weren't short of breath, and didn't feel cold all the time. While those on short daily HD were feeling better, those on standard in-center HD were feeling worse, and *losing function.* Given the choice, all of the people in the study chose to stay on short daily HD.[34]

Problems or Complications of Short Daily Home HD

Are there downsides of short daily HD? Yes. Some people tire of the routine and the time it takes to do set-up, clean-up, and deal with supplies. Travel with short daily HD is easier than it is with standard in-center HD—but not as easy as it was before kidney failure, or as it would be with a transplant.

In the short term, short daily home HD has a lot of pluses. The biggest drawback of short daily HD is in the long term. Short daily HD is a bit better at removing small wastes than standard in-center HD. It is not much better than standard in-center HD at clearing middle molecules like B2M out of your blood.[35] And, as you learned in Chapter 4, those middle molecules are the ones that can come back and bite you in the form of bone and joint damage. We find that people may start out on short daily HD and then switch to nocturnal. Or, some people do some short daily HD treatments and some nocturnal ones each week.

Survival with Short Daily HD

Two studies have looked at survival in short daily HD. One followed 26 people who switched from standard in-center HD to short daily. Survival over the four years of the study was 100%. In standard in-center HD, people spend an average of 14 days each year in the hospital.[36] Those in this study spent an average of just 1.25 days in the hospital. Another study pooled 23 years worth of data on 415 people who were on short daily HD for a total of 1,006 years. Although 20% of the people in this study died, this rate of survival was *2–3 times better than that of a matched group of U.S. people on standard in-center HD.* In fact, it was about the same as deceased donor transplant.[37]

Despite all of the benefits of short daily HD that you've read about in this chapter, some U.S. nephrologists insist that there really is no difference between short daily HD and standard in-center HD. They claim it's just that "better" (younger, smarter, more able to follow the treatment plan, healthier, etc...) people choose this treatment. And they would do just as well on any treatment. Not so! We know there is a real difference from studies that *follow the same people from standard in-center HD to short daily—and back again.*

Doctors are trained that the "gold standard" of research is the randomized, double-blind, placebo-controlled, crossover study. In case you're not a researcher, let's break that down:

- In a **randomized study**, people have an equal chance of landing in the control group (where things stay the same) and the experimental group (where things happen). Can we randomly assign people to a type of dialysis? Not really—no more than we could randomly assign them to smoke for 30 or 40 years and then see how many get cancer. All we can do is randomly assign those who would *agree* to do any type of dialysis.

- **Placebo-controlled** means that there is a fake treatment—like a sugar pill—and a real one. Is there such a thing as fake dialysis? Nope.

- A **double blind** study means that the researchers don't know who got the real vs. the fake treatment until the end of the study. This cannot be done with dialysis.

- **Crossover** means that people switch from one group to another. We *have* seen this. Many of the studies in this chapter have been crossovers from standard HD to short daily and sometimes back.

This "gold standard" type of study works quite well to test new drugs, but not as well for other things, like dialysis. We believe the evidence in favor of short daily HD speaks for itself. It's impossible to do a randomized study of dialysis, and there are no placebos here. What we have is *many* studies—that all point to the same conclusion: *more dialysis is more like having healthy kidneys.*

Here's a key point: we can't randomly assign people to get a kidney transplant or not, and see who lives longer. Yet we all seem to believe that people who get transplants live longer.

Wrapping Up Short Daily Home HD

If you want to feel good on a day-to-day basis—and perhaps improve your chance of longer survival—short daily home HD is a treatment you may want to do. It gives you nearly twice as much dialysis as you would get with standard in-center HD or even PD. More truly is better. Read on to find out why longer HD treatments are better yet.

Nocturnal Hemodialysis

When you choose nocturnal HD, you do your treatments at night while you sleep, for 7–8 hours. You can do nocturnal HD **at home** for up to 7 nights per week, or **in a clinic**, 3 nights per week. The more nights you do, the better you may feel. Even done three times per week nocturnal HD offers *twice* as much dialysis as standard HD—and far better removal of the middle molecules that cause long-term harm if they build up in your blood. And, since nocturnal HD treatments are done at night, they don't take time out of your day.

Nocturnal HD was the first type of chronic dialysis that was done in London in 1964 by Dr. Stanley Shaldon. So, it's not new, it's *back*. In the 1990s, a group in Humber River, Canada, including Drs. Robert Uldall, Andreas Pierratos, and David Mendelssohn, brought the option back to North America. When their reports came out about how much better people felt with so much HD, interest grew.

Dr. Robert Lockridge, a nephrologist from Lynchburg, VA, was concerned about a woman who had severe high blood pressure after 8 years of standard in-center HD. He went to Humber River in 1997 to learn the technique, and started a program in Lynchburg, that same year. (As of this writing, she is still doing nocturnal home HD 4 nights per week, works full-time, and has taken herself off of the transplant list—in 2011!) He's since published papers about nocturnal HD, done many talks, welcomed doctors from other clinics to learn nocturnal HD, and helped grow the treatment. His was nearly the only U.S. nocturnal HD program in 1997. Between 2004 and 2010, there has been 580% growth in the number of clinics that offer nocturnal home HD in the U.S. Today, there are nearly 500 that say they offer it. Australia brought back nocturnal HD in 2001, with government funding,[1] and found that it cost about 10% less than standard treatments.[2] Today, Australia does ten times as much nocturnal HD as the U.S., and has helped this option grow around the world.

Nocturnal HD treatments are very gentle and comfortable. Blood flow rates are slow, so nocturnal HD is easy on your access and your heart. Removal of wastes is *excellent*. Nocturnal HD done 5–6 nights per week replaces about 30% of kidney function. This is like turning back the clock to stage 3 CKD.[3]

How Nocturnal HD Works

Find a Nocturnal HD Clinic

To do nocturnal HD, you will need to find a clinic that offers it, and talk with your doctor. For information about how to find a clinic that offers nocturnal HD, see Chapter 8. The steps are the same for nocturnal HD as they are for short daily HD.

Nocturnal HD at Home

If you want to do nocturnal HD at home, most programs will require you to have a care partner who will train with you. Be sure to choose a clinic that has expertise in training people for this option. Read Chapter 12 to learn more. Of course, you'll be asleep—and so will your partner! Don't let anyone tell you that a partner must be awake—if someone says this, it is because lawyers are worried about lawsuits. Some nocturnal HD programs monitor treatments over the Internet. In practice, this does not seem to be any safer. Nocturnal HD is a very safe treatment on its own, because no other form of HD is more gentle. Read Chapters 8 and 10 to learn more about what we believe a care partner's ideal role is. (Hint: It involves *you* doing as much as possible yourself.)

Most people's biggest fear with nocturnal HD is having a needle pull out or the lines come apart when you're sleeping. Special safety steps are taken for nocturnal HD at home:

- You'll learn to tape the lines securely to reduce this risk.
- A Hemastrap® or T.N.T. Moborg *Immobilé* device can hold tubing in place on your arm so it doesn't kink or pull.[4] Or, some people use a lightweight sleeve that covers the needles and line connections.
- Some companies have a plastic clip that snaps over the line connection so it can't come apart.
- Bedwetting alarms have sensor pads that can be placed under the dialyzer *and* under the access arm. Even a single drop of blood will sound this type of alarm.
- A device made by Redsense uses an optical sensor at the access to detect any blood loss.

"Extended Hours" HD?

Some centers do not offer "nocturnal" HD, but they DO have what they call "extended hours" treatments. Why do they call it this? It's complicated.

The U.S. Food & Drug Administration (FDA) approves drugs and medical equipment, like HD machines. Once they approve a drug or machine, a doctor can prescribe it for *any* purpose. But, it can only be *marketed* (advertised) for the purpose given on the label. Any other use (by a doctor or a company) is "off-label." Off-label use of a product can lead to costly lawsuits if someone runs into trouble.

All dialysis machines on the market have been approved by the FDA. Right now, no machine is "FDA-approved" *for* nocturnal home HD; they are approved for in-center and home HD. Using an HD machine for nocturnal home HD is off-label. *This does not mean that nocturnal home HD is not safe*—people have been doing it for 50 years!

Nocturnal HD has been done safely for many years. We know of only two bleeding incidents. They were caught and stopped quickly. In both cases, bleeding was not from the access. It was from the connection of the tubing to the dialyzer (this is why it's wise to keep a bed wetting alarm under both the dialyzer *and* the access arm). Both people were okay.

Another concern of people who think about doing nocturnal HD is, "Will I be able to sleep?" Most do get used to doing their treatments while they sleep. If you have ever done PD with a cycler, it is quite similar. In some cases, it has taken people a few (cranky!) weeks to get the hang of being able to relax and sleep through a treatment. Covering the lights on the machine can help. One woman we know was only able to let go and fall asleep after she turned the front of the machine away from the bed so she couldn't see it. In Geelong, Australia, people hang a tea towel with the logo of the Geelong Cats (a mighty football team!) over the lights to hide them. You can be inventive—just be sure to run your thoughts past the training team to be sure there are no hidden risks to the solution you come up with. Tweak your set-up so you are comfortable and don't have to worry about pulling the lines. After you get things set, alarms will be less frequent, too.

Setting up a room for home nocturnal HD is a bit different than setting up for short daily HD. You don't need a chair, though some people do choose to use one. You may need to experiment a bit, but most people find that they prefer to use a bed. (Using a mattress protector or Chux® pad under your arm is wise, just in case.) Having a lot of clutter around can make it hard to sleep. You may want to find cupboards with doors or devote a closet to supplies so you don't have to see them on open shelves. Flooring is something to think about, too. Carpet is perhaps not the best choice in case there is a leak. A floor that looks nice and can be wiped off may work better for you.

If you do nocturnal HD at home, you may be able to do treatments 4–7 nights per week. This is the most dialysis now possible for you to get, and the most like having healthy kidneys. Medicare will routinely pay for 3 treatments per week. With a doctor's letter, they may pay for a 4th treatment. Some health plans will pay for more than 3 treatments per week, too.

Nocturnal HD in a Clinic

In-center nocturnal HD is growing very quickly in the U.S. For those who don't have a partner or who don't want to or can't do nocturnal HD at home, it may be the next best option. In-center nocturnal HD is also a great option during travel if you do home nocturnal. Three nights of treatment per week is twice as much HD as standard treatment—and it doesn't take time out of your day (or space out of your closet). Since the clinic is used for nocturnal treatments during off-hours, all of the other shifts must be done for the day. This means treatments tend to run from 8:00–9:00 p.m. until 4:00–5:00 a.m. so the morning crew can start at 6:00 a.m. This schedule can be a perfect fit if you're an early bird—but may not suit your body clock if you're a night owl.

Some people feel safer sleeping with in-center nocturnal HD, since they know the staff is there to keep an eye on them. **Just as with standard HD, it is still vital to never cover your access**. If a line does disconnect, you want to be sure the staff can see it. In-center HD is most often done in the same chairs the clinic uses during the day. If these bother you for 4 hours, they may be a real problem for 8. You might ask about bringing in an eggshell cushion to see if that will help. The treatments themselves are *much* more comfortable—you should not have cramps, headaches, etc. with any type of nocturnal HD. A sleep mask and earplugs (or perhaps an iPod with quiet music) can help you tune out the others in the room. The staff will dim the lights, but can't turn them off, because they need to be able to see you.

When you have a partner, it can be odd not to sleep in your own bed 3 nights each week. One woman we knew really missed her husband of 50 years when he did nocturnal HD in-center. They switched to home nocturnal, and, last we heard, were doing very well.

The Nocturnal HD Machine

When your treatments last 8 hours, the few minutes of prep time seem to be less of a bother for some people. Nocturnal can be done using any HD machine that is on the market, like the Fresenius 2008K@home™. A full-size machine may need to have complex water treatment. At home, this means having a place near your plumbing to put one or two carbon or reverse osmosis tanks, often a bathroom or basement. (New machines are being designed right now that will have water treatment built in.) Your training nurse must then teach you how to use more equipment.

Nocturnal Home HD Training

When you plan to do nocturnal HD at home, you'll have a home visit. This is not to judge you. The home training nurse will help you figure out where to put the machine and supplies so your set-up will work best for you and your partner. If you'll use a standard machine, your home will need plumbing and wiring changes. Some clinics will pay for these; others will charge you for them. Medicare expects clinics to pay for minor changes that are needed. In most cases, the updates cost in the range of $1,500 or less. A technician will guide an electrician and a plumber so the changes are done right.

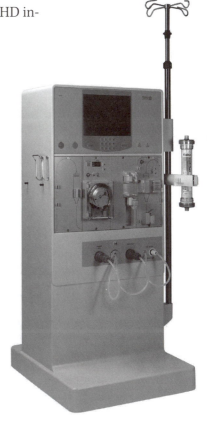

Fresenius 2008K@home™
Photo permission of Fresenius
Medical Care – North America

In most cases, you and a partner will start to train for nocturnal HD during the day. You'll learn about the machine, blood tests, trouble shooting, needle placement, how to order supplies, and all of the other steps. You'll do shorter (4-6 hour) treatments with the training nurse on hand for at least a week or two, or until you are *confident* in the machine and in yourself. Your blood test results will be checked to keep track of when you need to cut back on (or stop) blood pressure pills and phosphate binders. Do make the jump to nights, though. The longer, gentler treatments you can get are worth it.

Once you can show that you know how to set up and use the machine, you may do some shorter treatments at night in the clinic or at a hospital. Your training nurse will want to be sure that you will wake up if an alarm goes off (he or she will set some off on purpose so you can practice). If you have hearing or vision problems, this is a chance to set you up with an assist device or special alarm and test how well it works for you. Then you may do a few full-length treatments at night, still in the clinic. Be sure to ask how to disconnect if you need to go to the bathroom, since this will happen at home.

When you do go home, you may want to start out by doing your treatments during the *day* until you're used to being in the new setting. Things can seem scarier at night, and daylight can help ease your mind. Your home training nurse may come and watch your first treatment at home. A nurse will be on call by phone, any time, to help you through the questions you're sure to have. You may call often in the first few weeks. After that, you'll start to find that you can handle most things on your own, and ask questions during your monthly clinic visits.

As with short daily HD training (see Chapter 8), prepare to be overwhelmed at first! Even if you've done short daily treatments, and are going home with the same machine, there is still a lot more to learn—and some things to unlearn. Plan to clear your schedule and make things easy on yourself, so you don't have too much going on. You want to be able to devote yourself to learning nocturnal HD without being too stressed out by other things in your life. It can help you to know up front that there will be times when you feel like you'll never get it, it's too much. Show your care partner that you appreciate him or her, too. How? Here's what one care partner said:

"Pay attention to the little ways you can help ease the load for your care partner. Most of the time and attention is on the patient, so when he asks me how I'm doing and what can he do to help me, that means a lot. We also have our own medical problems that need care and sometimes we don't have time to tend to our own needs, whether it is our own doctor visits, or time for exercise, enough sleep, etc. If I don't take care of myself, then I can't be a good caregiver for my hubby, but it's hard to find time.

So, do all you can for yourself during treatment so your care partner can relax at least a little. During the rest of the time, run errands or do all you can around the house so the care partner doesn't have to try to do everything.

Today my sweetie had put some wrapped chocolates in his pocket before dialysis. Just after I got him on the machine, he reached over, held my hand and put the chocolate in my hand and said, "thanks for all you do for me." That means so much and was a nice surprise!"

Who Can Do Nocturnal HD

Anyone who needs dialysis would benefit from doing nocturnal HD, at home or in the clinic. It's simply more dialysis, which is more like having healthy kidneys! Since "anyone" (well, nearly anyone) seems to be suited for standard in-center HD, it's hard to think of a reason why anyone would *not* be suited for in-center nocturnal HD. As long as you can have an access, it should be possible to do nocturnal treatments. People who have trouble with gaining and removing too much fluid on standard in-center HD and have blood pressure drops will feel *much* better on in-center nocturnal HD.

The choice of going *home* with nocturnal HD is a bigger one. Getting over the "hump" of doing treatments while you're asleep can take some time and some confidence that you may not have at the start. We find that in the U.S., many people tend to start out with standard in-center HD or PD and then switch to short daily. After they find out how much better they can feel with daily fluid removal, they see that nocturnal could make them feel even better—and would take less time out of their day. Plus, they know that they can do the steps of the treatment and handle any glitches that arise. In Australia, there is no short daily HD at this time, so people go right to nocturnal HD, and they do fine with it.

Steven's Story: Nocturnal Home HD

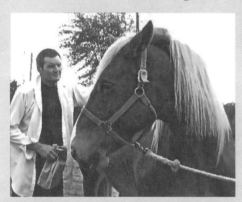

In March of 1979, when I was 29, my kidney disease reached the point where I needed dialysis. Since I have Alport's Syndrome, and my mother and brother were home hemo patients, it wasn't really a surprise.

At first, for a very short time, I did dialyze in a clinic after getting off work. I was sometimes late getting there, the staff was late getting others off the machine, and it just wasn't working for me. Shortly after that I went on home HD with a Drake-Willock machine, to give me more schedule flexibility. I learned of a Gambro machine—the first one with a heat disinfect mode. Convinced that this could improve the machine cleaning, I started to look into it. My clinic was against bringing in any outside machine. With my nephrologists' support, I got the new machine, against the wishes of the clinic administrator.

Gambro is a Swedish company. They sent a tech over from Sweden to assemble stacks of boxes into a machine. The tech told us that in Europe, nearly everyone on home hemo did their treatments at *night*, so they could keep their jobs during the day. We were always late getting on, so this sounded like a good idea. I worked full time and had always had an exercise program. After talking with my doctor, (who had gone to medical school in England, and was very familiar with the value and safety of dialyzing at night), my wife and I got started. I felt much better.

Nocturnal treatments let both me and my wife keep working full time, and allowed me to keep up regular exercise—jogging on non-treatment days before work. Since going 2 days between treatments can be a little exhausting, my nephrologist recommended that we try an every other night schedule to get rid of the big shifts in fluid and clearances after two days. Then, not only did I feel better, I kept a more even weight gain between treatments.

After 10 years, the Gambro needed to be upgraded to an AK-10 model. This one came with Bicarb, which really made a difference in what I felt like doing. I went back to grad school, got an MBA, moved back to a modest ranch, and started a cattle operation, plus my full-time job. Ten years later, that machine was getting to be a maintenance nightmare and was harder to get repaired. This meant sometimes I had to run in-center, which totally disrupted our work schedules. Gambro got out of the home HD business in the USA, so we were switched to a Seratron. After all this time with Gambro, which seemed to run well until the 9-10 year mark, the Seratron was a disappointment. Baxter took over, and replaced that with a Tina, which also wasn't as reliable as what we had become accustomed to.

Baxter told us in late 2008 that they were getting out of the home hemo business and would soon no longer support the machine. We began the search for a new one. And, Medicare announced that they were getting rid of Method 2. We looked at two home clinics in our town. In June of 2009, I started checking what options were available. The first one was a NxStage only (short daily treatments) clinic, though they did advertise that they had all options for home hemo. I had been dialyzing for 7 hours, every other night for nearly 30 years, and a nightly short run was not very appealing. By this time, I had started two companies and continued to operate a modest cattle ranch. My day starts at 5:30, and often doesn't end until 10 pm. There are times I need to be out of town for business, or as hobbyist, showing dogs in conformation. I didn't think I would feel as well, and was worried about being able to get enough time on dialysis. In my time on home HD, I have never needed meds for blood pressure, and have always run a Hct/Hbg of 47-55%/16-17g/dL. I have never had a dialysis related hospitalization. My fistula was revised one time, 15 years out, with no problems since. I feel like longer, slower dialysis is one of the reasons.

We learned that there was a home hemo machine, the Fresenius 2008K2. We finally got one in January of 2010.

Now, I ride my bicycle 12-14 miles every morning before work, and still work full time. I never would have been able to keep working or feel as good as I do without this type of dialysis.

Your Lifestyle on Nocturnal HD

We said in the intro of this book that your choice of a treatment option would affect every aspect of your lifestyle. In the case of nocturnal HD, here's how:

Time Commitment

Most nocturnal HD treatments last about 8 hours, plus set-up and clean-up time. All in all, your weekly hours would look like this:

Table 9-1: Time commitment for Nocturnal HD

Task	Time	Number of Treatments	Total
HD treatment	8 hours	3 – 6	24-48
Set-up/Clean-up (OR travel to and from a clinic)	45 min	3 – 6	2.25 – 4.5 hours
Recovery time to feel well again	10 min[5]	3 – 6	30 min to 1 hour
			26.7 to 53.5 hours

Besides the 26.75 to 53.5 hours for treatments, set-up and clean-up (or clinic travel time), and recovery, you'll need to plan time once a month for a clinic visit, and to order, receive, and put away supplies. Of course, *only the set-up, clean-up, clinic visit, and supply hours are during the day*. The rest of nocturnal HD is done at night while you sleep.

When you do nocturnal HD at home, and have a care partner, he or she can sleep, too. So, nocturnal HD will take less time out of his or her day, too, than some other options. It is vital that one of you be able to wake up quickly if there is an alarm, and react to fix the problem. You will practice this during training, and won't go home until you and the training nurse are sure that you will be safe.

In-center nocturnal HD will give you about 24 hours of treatment per week during the night, plus travel time to and from the clinic. So, in terms of time *out of your day*, nocturnal HD at home or in-center takes the least of any type of dialysis—while giving you two to four times as much treatment. This is the best HD time bargain you can get.

How You'll Feel During and After Treatment

Nocturnal HD treatments themselves should not hurt. With a fistula or a graft, you'll use needles. Most people who do nocturnal HD and have a fistula use the Buttonhole technique to make the needle placement nearly painless (see page 50). Since you'll be asleep, you may not even notice much about the treatment, unless an alarm goes off. Long, slow, nocturnal treatments won't cause your blood pressure to drop,[6] so you do not have to keep the dialysate cold to control low blood pressure. That means *you* won't feel cold during dialysis—a common complaint with standard in-center HD.

We just said that your blood pressure won't drop on nocturnal HD. It turns out that there may be more than one reason for this. One reason, of course, is that the treatment is slow and gentle. But also, it turns out that having your blood outside of your body in clear plastic tubing during the day means that it is *exposed to light*. In an HD clinic, these lights tend to be fluorescent tubes, which have wavelengths that are known to have an effect on living cells. A study was done of 10 people on standard HD.[7] For one week, half of their treatments were done as usual. During other the half, the dialyzer and lines were covered with aluminium foil to shield them from the light. Those who had the shielding had much lower levels of *nitric oxide* (NO). NO can trigger episodes of low blood pressure. So, if you do your treatments at night, you may also be protecting your blood vessels from the ill effects of too much light.

Eating and Drinking

When your treatment does two to four times the work of standard HD, you don't have to do as much yourself. With nocturnal HD, this means you won't have strict limits on fluid, sodium, phosphorus, and potassium. Nocturnal HD removes more than twice as much phosphorus as standard HD[8]—*so much that some people need phosphate supplements!* Calcium-phosphate product was lower,[9] which means there is less risk of growing bone where you don't want it (*extraskeletal calcification*). Your target levels for nutrients will be based on how many nights per week you do treatments, and whether you have a 2-day gap (as with in-center nocturnal HD). Your dietitian will work with your doctor to track your blood tests and make any diet adjustments you need.

Nocturnal HD also seems to improve appetite so you *want* to eat. A study of 14 people followed for 1–2 years on nocturnal HD found that their appetite, body weight, energy level, and protein intake all improved.[10] Their phosphate levels stayed in the target range without binders, too. In Australia, it is common that once people feel better and eat better, they gain "real" (not water) weight. This means that your dry weight will need to be tweaked. How will you know this is happening? Your blood pressures before and after dialysis will slowly start to drop.

With nocturnal HD, you can go out with friends or have dinner with family and eat and drink pretty much as they do! Many social outings center around food. Feeling "normal" and not having to make special requests can help remove some of the burden of kidney failure for you.

That said, we hope you'll use your new freedom to add in more nuts, fresh fruit and veggies, and protein—not just cheese and chocolate and colas. Each cell in your body is made out of the foods you eat, so healthy choices can help you feel your best.

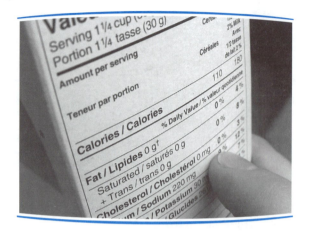

Avoid *trans fats*—fats made solid for a longer shelf life by injecting hydrogen. These fake fats can:[11]

- Trigger inflammation throughout your body
- Increase harmful fat around your organs
- Cause insulin resistance
- Damage your heart

Trans fats are mainly found in grain products—from bread and bagels to cookies and pie crusts. Look for "Zero Trans" on the front of food packages. Read the labels, too, and if you see the words "partially hydrogenated," or "interesterified" (a new type of oil that may be even worse than trans fats), look for a better choice.

Medications

One of the first reports about nocturnal HD from Canada found that fewer (or no) blood pressure pills were needed and people no longer had to take phosphate binders.[12] If you no longer needed just these two drugs, it might mean as many as 20 fewer pills to take—and pay for—each day.

People who do nocturnal HD may also need lower doses of costly anemia drugs. One study compared 32 people using standard in-center HD to 63 who switched from standard in-center HD to nocturnal HD. At the start, both groups had the same levels of hemoglobin (Hb) and iron, and were on the same EPO dose. By 12 months later, the nocturnal group had much better Hb levels—with less EPO.[13] Other studies have found the same thing.[14] Why? Red blood cells are alive, with a lifespan of about 4 months. But if your blood is a toxic soup, your red blood cells won't live as long. On nocturnal HD, the blood is much cleaner, so red blood cells live longer. A study was done of the plasma of people before and after they switched from standard in-center HD to nocturnal HD. In the nocturnal HD plasma, the "progenitor" cells that grow into red blood cells grew much better than they did in the standard in-center HD plasma.[15] Cleaner blood for your cells is like cleaner water and air for you—just a better, more healthy place to live.

These are some of the types of drugs that are common for people on nocturnal HD:

- **Cholesterol medications** – to help prevent damage to your heart.
- **Cinacalcet (Sensipar®)** – to help treat too-high levels of parathyroid hormone that can cause bone disease.
- **Erythropoiesis stimulating agents (ESAs)** – injections to treat anemia (a shortage of red blood cells) by making more red blood cells. Treating anemia can give you more energy and help prevent heart damage. People on nocturnal HD may need lower doses.
- **Iron** – to provide the building blocks to make red blood cells.
- **Renal vitamins** – with kidney failure, "normal" vitamins could build up to toxic levels.
- **Vitamin D** – to help your body use calcium better and help avoid bone problems.

Working

Any type of treatment that you can do at night while you sleep makes it easier to hold a day job. And a treatment that lets you eat normal food, feel better, and have more energy is a great fit for work. Nocturnal HD is the very *definition* of work-friendly!

It's also tough to be on the job when you're in the hospital. On nocturnal HD, hospital stays are far less common. A study compared 32 people on nocturnal HD to 42 people on standard in-center HD. For the people on standard in-center HD, the rate of hospital days stayed the same during the 2 years of the study. But those who switched to nocturnal HD had three times fewer hospital days—and they were mainly for access, not heart, problems.[16]

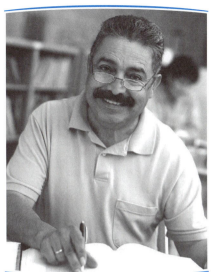

Travel

When you do home nocturnal HD with a standard machine or you do in-center nocturnal HD, you may want to seek out an in-center nocturnal program when you travel. In-center nocturnal HD can be tricky to find. There are not as many clinics that offer it. Ask your social worker if he or she has a list of clinics owned by the same company that owns your clinic. You can also check the "Find a Clinic" database on Home Dialysis Central (www.homedialysis.org), but this list is not complete—there may be others.

CAUTION: *If you switch to standard in-center HD when you travel, be very careful about what you eat.* It's easy to get used to the freedom of eating what you like—like tomatoes, dried fruit, mangos, avocados, and other high potassium treats. But we know of a man who did in-center nocturnal HD at one of the first clinics that offered it. He was doing quite well—until he went to Florida on vacation and overdid the tropical fruits. Sadly, he died. Talk to your dietitian before you go, so you can eat safely and have a good trip.

Exercise

If you like to be active, nocturnal HD is a good choice. We bet you won't be surprised to learn that nocturnal HD aids the ability to exercise. A study followed 13 people on standard in-center HD who switched to nocturnal HD. Their exercise was measured before the switch, and then 2 months and 3–6 months after. At each step, they were able to exercise longer and harder than they'd done before.[17]

Body Image

There are no studies on this topic that we could find, but we can tell you that people who switch from standard in-center HD to nocturnal HD *look better*. Their skin is a healthy color. Their eyes are bright. They have more energy. The itching, rashes, and other skin problems that are common with standard in-center HD are much less so with nocturnal HD.

Intimacy

"You can't get too much sex, too much religion, or too much dialysis," Dr. John Bower, from Mississippi, likes to say—and that was before nocturnal HD came back on the scene. When you feel better all around—and more like yourself—your sex life is likely to improve. Just being able to do your usual roles in your family can help you feel more worthwhile and valued. Not being "the sick one" matters! As we said in Chapter 8 on short daily HD, if a lower libido or erectile problems are due to the disease that made your kidneys fail, they won't go away, and there are other options for you. But, if loss of desire or other problems are due to poor treatment, nocturnal HD can change your life.

In a very small study done at WellBound (a dialysis company that trains and supports many people on home HD), 11 people were followed from standard to short daily HD and then nocturnal HD.[18] At each point they were asked to rate their sex lives on a scale of 1 to 10, with 10 being best. Here are their ratings on each option:

- **Standard in-center HD: 1.6 (out of 10)**
- **Short daily HD: 4.4 (out of 10)**
- **Nocturnal HD: 9.2 (out of 10)**

There are not very many people yet who have tried all three HD options. So, while these numbers are very small, it's good to keep in mind that no one knows what a treatment is really like unless they try it. Those who took part in this study clearly had better sexual function on nocturnal HD than they had before.

You may have to be a bit creative about where and when to be intimate when you do your treatments in your bed. Of course, there is always before or after treatment. Once you start a treatment, you'd need to be very careful of the lines and needles, but it could be done. Other rooms and other times can work, as well.

Fertility

Nocturnal HD gives you about as much kidney replacement as a transplant—but without drugs to suppress the immune system. So, it makes sense that nocturnal HD would make it more possible to get pregnant and have a baby than other forms of dialysis, though there are no large studies. In one case report, a 31 year old woman whose blood pressure would not come down on standard in-center HD switched to nocturnal HD 5-6 nights per week. Eight months later, she started to have normal menstrual cycles again. Two years after starting nocturnal HD, she became pregnant. Her prescription was raised to 7 nights per week, and she had a healthy baby.[19]

As we said in Chapter 6, researchers in Canada found five women in one region who wanted to have babies and were on HD. While they did standard in-center HD, none got pregnant. After they switched to nocturnal HD, they had seven pregnancies among them, and gave birth to six babies. Two were small for gestational age, and one was a preemie (less than 32 weeks).[20]

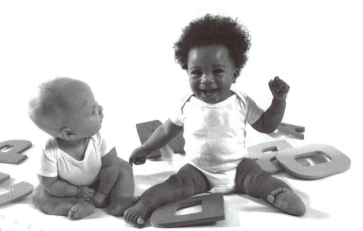

This study does *not* tell us how many women wanted to get pregnant but were not able to. And, it doesn't tell us how much of a challenge it was to care for an infant when you do nocturnal HD. If you choose to try, you'll want to think through the logistics and figure out what you'll do when the baby cries at night.

Sleep

You might think that it would be hard to sleep with your blood outside of your body—and this is a problem for some people, at least at first. But if you can get past that, studies find that sleep quality is *better* on nocturnal HD than on other types of HD.

Melatonin is a hormone that helps control sleep rhythm. In a study that compared people on standard in-center HD, cycler PD, and nocturnal HD, those who did standard in-center HD had the worst sleep. People who did nocturnal HD had a normal rise in melatonin level at night, while the others did not.[21]

As many as 50% of people on standard in-center HD may have *sleep apnea* (a problem where breathing stops many times during the night).[22] One reason for sleep apnea on standard in-center HD may be that the throat actually narrows inside because it swells due to excess water in the blood. A study of 24 people who switched from standard in-center HD to nocturnal HD found that their throats became larger again on nocturnal HD.[23]

Good sleep itself is linked with longer life on dialysis. In a study of 11,351 people on standard in-center HD from 7 different countries, nearly half said they slept poorly. Those who slept poorly had a 16% higher risk of death. Better dialysis means better sleep.

Benefits of Nocturnal HD

Better Fluid Removal

Did you happen to read Chapter 6? In it, we told you why blood pressure drops, cramps, headaches, nausea, and just all around feeling awful are so common after standard in-center HD. A standard in-center HD treatment can pull fluid out of your blood (ultrafiltration rate, or UFR) faster than your body can keep up with. How you feel in the short term, from day to day, on HD is *entirely* about how much fluid is removed and how quickly. It can take *years* to feel the effects of poor waste removal, but you can feel fluid removal the same day.

So, what if your treatment is *twice* as long—8 hours? Look what happens in Table 9-2. As you can see, now blood volume is much more stable. With nocturnal HD, a lower UFR can be used—*even with much more fluid to remove*. This means fewer (or no) symptoms for you. Cramps, vomiting, and feeling dizzy or wiped out after a treatment just *do not happen*.

As it turns out, even laying flat for a treatment, since most people do nocturnal treatments in a bed, can help you get a better treatment. When you sit up, gravity pulls fluid into your legs. There is less water in your blood, and more in between your cells. When you lie down, water in your tissues seeps back into your bloodstream.[24]

Table 9-2: Eight hour dialysis treatments

HD time (Hrs)	Water gain in mL	UFR	Rate of water refill from interstitium	Change in blood volume	Chance of symptoms or BP drop
8	800 mL	100 mL/hr	100 mL/hr	0	0
8	1600 mL	200 mL/hr	200 mL/hr	0	0
8	2400 mL	300 mL/hr	300 mL/hr	0	0
8	3200 mL	400 mL/hr	400 mL/hr	0	0
8	4800 mL	600 mL/hr	400 mL/hr	- 200 mL/hr	Small

Better water removal has a whole host of benefits for you. On nocturnal HD, the *mean arterial pressure*—average BP in a day—was much lower than it was on standard in-center HD.[25] This puts less stress on your heart.[26] After people with congestive heart failure switched from standard in-center to nocturnal HD, their hearts got stronger and they needed fewer heart drugs.[27] Switching to nocturnal HD also made the blood vessels more sensitive to changes in heart rate and blood volume—in other words, more like the blood vessels of healthy people.[28]

UFR rates can be quite low with nocturnal HD—and blood flow rates (BFR) are far lower as well. Often, treatments run at a blood flow rate of 200 to 300 mL/min. This may be only 40% to 50% as fast as standard in-center HD blood flows. Slower blood flows are a plus for your heart—and your access. We suspect that one reason Japan and Europe have much higher fistula rates is that they do even their standard treatments more slowly, at about 300 mL/min., rather than the 400 to 500 mL/min. that is common in the U.S.

Left ventricular hypertrophy (LVH), as we've said, is a leading cause of death for people on dialysis. This overgrowth of the heart's main pumping chamber leads to heart failure or sudden death. It is very common for people who have been on standard in-center HD to have some degree of LVH. A study compared 28 people on nocturnal HD to 13 people doing standard HD at home who had similar ages, blood pressure, LVH, and hemoglobin levels. After 2 years, the group doing standard HD at home had no changes. But the nocturnal HD group had much lower blood pressure, took fewer blood pressure pills, and had *less* LVH. *Their hearts were healthier.*[29] A second study randomly assigned 52 people to either do standard in-center HD three times per week or nocturnal HD six nights per week. By 6 months later, the standard HD group's left ventricles were a little *bigger*—but the nocturnal HD group's were *much smaller.* Their blood pressure was lower, too. Those doing nocturnal HD had fewer symptoms and felt like their disease and treatment were less of a burden than those on standard in-center HD.[30]

Blood vessels in other parts of the body may be helped by nocturnal HD, too. A 42 year old man had started standard in-center HD in 1976. He switched to nocturnal HD because he had painful peripheral artery disease. He also had soft tissue calcification in his hands, legs, and back. On nocturnal HD, he became "symptom free"—and had better blood flow to his legs.[31]

Better Waste Removal

As we said, how you feel from one day to the next on dialysis is *all* about fluid removal: how much and how fast. But in the long-term, what matters to your blood vessels, bones, joints, nerves, and tissues is *waste removal*. Wastes that build up in your blood can poison you in many ways (read in Chapter 4). Apart from transplant, nocturnal HD is your best bet to remove wastes and protect yourself down the road.

Below, in Table 9-3, you can see the results of a computer model that looks at how well standard in-center HD, short daily HD, and three times a week nocturnal HD remove five different substances.[32]

Table 9-3: Waste Removal Rates with Standard HD, Short Daily HD, and Nocturnal HD

Substance	Standard HD	Short Daily HD	Nocturnal HD (3x/week)
Urea	12.5*	14.61 (+16.9% over standard HD)	19.49 (+ 55.9% over standard HD)
Creatinine	10.16	11.73 (+15.5%)	17.04 (**+ 67.7%**)
Vitamin B$_{12}$	6.29	7.30 (+16.1%)	11.34 (**+ 80.3%**)
Inulin	3.47	3.65 (+ 5.2%)	6.00 (**+ 72.9%**)
B2M	4.74	4.86 (+ 2.5%)	6.18 (**+ 30.4%**)

All wastes are reported in milliliters removed per minute of treatment.

It is easy to see that waste removal is far better with nocturnal HD—and that's just with three treatments per week. Four or five or six treatments are even better.

Better waste removal means a cleaner climate for all of your cells. This may be one reason why people who switched from standard in-center HD had far more active vitamin D in their blood after 6 months of nocturnal HD.[33] (Better phosphate removal is a second reason.) The middle molecule interleukin-6 (IL-6) stops your bone marrow from making more red blood cells. Nocturnal HD removes more IL-6, which may explain why hemoglobin levels are higher with less EPO.[34]

Though doctors are not sure why, nocturnal HD seems to improve lipid (fat) levels in the blood, too. People on standard in-center HD tend to have high levels of triglycerides and other fats that can harm the blood vessels and heart. In 11 people who switched from standard to nocturnal HD, these fat levels were far lower just 3 months later.[35]

Less Calcification

You really don't want your blood vessels to be like stone. They are meant to be supple, so they can flex in response to changes in blood volume or pressure. Nocturnal HD—even 3 nights per week—improved blood vessel calcification in a study of 26 people who switched from standard home HD. One year later, 90% did not need phosphate binders. Their bones stayed just as dense, but their PTH and calcium-phosphate products both dropped. And 87.5% had blood vessels that were less calcified, or had not gotten any worse.[36]

Besides the blood vessels, a rare problem with dialysis is lumps of calcium-phosphate that can form anywhere in the body. One man had calcium tumors in his shoulder, hands, and feet. Even short daily HD did not help. But his hard to control phosphate levels went back to normal after a week of nocturnal HD. And 9 months after starting nocturnal HD *the tumors melted away*.[37]

Clearer Thinking

Kidney failure can cause fuzzy thinking or trouble focusing. On standard in-center HD, people report just not feeling as mentally sharp as they once did. Does more dialysis help? It might. In a small pilot study, 12 people switched from standard to nocturnal HD. They were each given ten tests to measure their thinking skills and emotional state. After 6 months, they had 22% fewer cognitive symptoms, were thinking 7% faster, and had 32% better attention and working memory.[38]

Problems or Complications of Nocturnal HD

One of the biggest pluses of nocturnal HD is being able to do treatments at night while you sleep. And one of the biggest challenges is...getting used to doing treatments at night while you sleep. There is no question that this can sound easier than it really is in practice. People who get over the hurdle *love* nocturnal HD so much that some have taken themselves off of the transplant list. They feel great, eat a normal diet, and don't want to rock the boat by taking drugs to suppress their immune system. Others grab that transplant brass ring as soon as it comes by.

In both the short and long term, nocturnal HD has far more pluses than minuses. One concern that some people have noted is the extra exposure to plastic. Phthalates are chemicals used to make plastic soft and flexible so it can be used for things like tubing and bags. They are also linked with an increased cancer risk. All dialysis exposes you to some type of plastic. Most of the studies of phthalates have been done in animals, but some companies do make dialysis supplies without them. Still, with nocturnal HD, your blood is in contact with the dialyzer and lines longer than it is with other treatments. It's hard to say what impact this might have—but we doubt it overcomes the benefits of this treatment. You will have to weigh the benefits and risks.

Survival with Nocturnal HD

As we said at the start of this chapter, nocturnal HD is not new, it's *back*. In Tassin, France, Dr. Bernard Charra[39] gave people 8-hour long treatments for *30 years*. His papers report some of the best HD outcomes in the world:

- **87% of those who dialyzed at his clinic were alive at 5 years**
- **75% were alive at 10 years**
- **55% were alive at 15 years**
- **43% were alive at 20 years**

With standard in-center HD in the U.S., the overall mortality rate is about 20% *each year*. Of course, as you saw in Chapter 6, this varies a lot by age and health. But it means that Dr. Charra's long treatments were truly life-saving.

One study used data from two Canadian programs and the U.S.[40] Researchers used a random process to match each of 177 people who did nocturnal HD to *three* people who'd had kidney transplants. They followed all 1,239 people for up to 12 years. During the study, 14.7% of those on nocturnal HD died. This was just a hair more than the 14.3% who had deceased donor transplants—a statistical dead heat. Survival with nocturnal HD was *just the same* as deceased donor transplant. Living donor transplants do tend to do better. They did better in this study, too—only 8.5% of people who'd had a living donor transplant died during the 12 years of the study.

Another study matched each of 94 people who did nocturnal HD to *ten* people using standard HD. This study also found significantly fewer hospital days and higher survival in those who did nocturnal treatments.[41] WHY do people seem to live longer on nocturnal HD? A study compared 87 people using nocturnal HD with the rest of the US dialysis population. The researchers found that two things mattered: education level and hours of treatment time.[42]

One thing we wonder about is how much better survival on nocturnal HD would be if people *would give it a try sooner*. In the U.S., most people start on standard in-center HD, then some go to SDHD, and finally a brave few go on to nocturnal HD. But each year of standard in-center HD can raise the risk of long-term damage. If you are on standard in-center HD and thinking of going home—on any treatment—we applaud you! Sooner is better than later, but later is much better than not at all.

Wrapping Up Nocturnal HD

In this chapter you've learned that nocturnal HD does a superb job of removing fluid—and wastes. It takes much less time out of the day but delivers more than twice as much treatment for your effort. On it, you can eat a normal diet, drink more fluids—and take fewer drugs.

Why don't more people do nocturnal HD, if it's so great? Good question. In Canada, researchers asked people on standard in-center HD why they didn't want to do nocturnal HD. Here are the reasons they gave:

- They didn't think they could do the treatments.
- They didn't think they could put in their own needles.
- They'd been on standard in-center HD and it was what they were used to.
- They were afraid of being a burden to their partners.
- They worried about something going wrong.[43]

If you have seen the Home Dialysis Central website (www.homedialysis.org), you know that we use Dorothy from the Wizard of Oz movie as an icon. Just looking at it, you think, "*there's no place like home*." And it's true! It's also true that anything worth having is worth fighting for. *A good life is worth fighting for*. But, like the Cowardly Lion, you need courage. You need to believe in yourself and know that you can do it. We believe in you.

And, we believe in your partner. In Chapter 10, we'll talk about partner roles in home dialysis, and what works best.

The Care Partner's Role in Home Dialysis

We use the term "*care partner*" on purpose in this chapter. Often, the word that's used is "*caregiver*." That may be a good fit if someone needs a *lot* of help with care. In fact, though, we find that there are two groups of people who do home dialysis:

1. *Most* people who do home treatment are pretty healthy other than their kidney failure, regardless of age. They may have diabetes, or even have had a heart attack or two, but they can think and learn and move well. They want to work or travel or have a life. They want to be able to eat better, take fewer meds, and improve their chance of living longer.

2. A far smaller group of people on home dialysis is **very ill**, may be bed or chair bound, and needs quite a lot of care. We've heard of children with complex genetic problems, people who've had strokes, who need breathing tubes, or families who want to care for a beloved but frail loved one at home after seeing how poorly they feel on standard HD.

We wrote this chapter for people who are thinking about helping a **pretty healthy person** do a home treatment for kidney failure. The issues of being an all-around *caregiver* for someone who is very ill are beyond the scope of this book. Other books and websites do a good job with things like burnout and finding a way to get some time for yourself. We'll list some in Chapter 14.

Your Role in Standard In-center HD

The person you're thinking of helping with home dialysis may be new to dialysis. But most often, people start out with standard HD in a center or PD and then may switch to a home HD option after days, months, or years. When this is the case, you might worry that be-ing a care partner for home dialysis will be a lot of work for you, when you "weren't doing anything" with standard HD. After all, the clinic staff did the treatments, and you may not have had any role in them.

Often, though, people who don't feel well on standard HD may not do all of the things they used to do. This can put quite a *large* burden on you. For example, you might:

- **Work more** (or live on less income) because the person on standard HD doesn't feel well enough to work full-time and has gone on disability or retired early.

- **Do more of the cooking**—and the clean up—because he or she may feel too wiped out after a treatment to do it. And, you may be cooking two meals: one with less salt, potassium, and phosphorus and one "normal" one.

- **Mow the lawn or shovel snow** (or pay someone to do it), or do more of the garden work.

- **Run more errands**, like taking the car to the shop or the kids to the doctor or the cat to the vet.

- **Cancel family trips, concerts, reunions, or even dinners out** with friends at the last minute, because he or she is too tired or sick to go. Or, go by yourself.

- **Miss intimacy** with a partner who has less interest in sex.

- **Help cope with losses** of others who dialyzed in-center and passed away—perhaps at treatment—or with other upsetting events that occur in the center.

Helping someone to do home dialysis may well end up to be *less* of a burden on you than standard in-center HD is if he or she can take back some of the roles they used to do before. Your day to day role as a care partner of a pretty healthy person on home dialysis can range from quite small to quite large, depending on what you work out together. Kidney failure on its own should not make people so sick that they can't take an active role in their own care. (Poorly done standard in-center HD can have this effect on some people. As more treatment is done during home training, your loved one should start to feel much better.) So, we strongly urge a pretty healthy person to do as many of the tasks related to home treatment as possible. It's his or her treatment, after all, not yours.

Types of Home Dialysis

How much work you might do as the partner of someone on home dialysis will depend on which type of treatment he or she does. You can read about the treatments in Chapters 6–9.

- **Manual PD** – People who do manual PD don't need to have a care partner if they can manage on their own. If you are married or in a relationship with someone who does PD, you may have no role at all. Or, you might choose to take on a role. For example, if you're very organized and like to keep track of things, you might keep a list of supplies that will be needed. Or, you might take and record blood pressure readings. If your loved one can't lift the PD bags, you may have a role hanging them up for each exchange. If you are strong and able to carry boxes of fluid, you might open a new box and put the bags where they'll be needed. Some early risers will heat up a bag for a person on PD, so it's ready to go for the morning exchange.

- **Cycler PD** – No partner is required for PD with a cycler. If you sleep in the same room as someone who does cycler PD, you may or may not choose to take on a role. (But you will hear the alarms.) Cycler bags are heavier than manual ones, so the person on PD may need your help to lift them up onto the cycler. In Canada, there is a program where nurses come to the homes of older people who use PD and connect them to the cycler. In the morning the nurses come back and unhook them. In this way, older people can stay in their homes instead of going to a clinic for HD. We don't know of anything like this in the U.S., but some health plans may offer it. Ask! Helping someone to do PD may be less of a burden than driving to and from a clinic three times per week.

- **Standard Home HD** – We don't suggest this option today for two reasons. First, standard HD (3–4 hour treatments, three days a week with a 2-day no-treatment gap) is just not as good as more dialysis. And second, standard HD at home has a very high care partner burden. The chance of running into the types of problems that often occur in-center, like low blood pressure and cramps, is high. This option can give your loved one more dialysis than standard in-center HD, though, if short daily or nocturnal HD are not yet offered where you live. Some people choose to do longer treatments with standard home HD, or dialyze every other day to get rid of the 2-day no-treatment gap. In fact, most short daily and nocturnal home HD programs in the U.S. still require a care partner today because they have not adjusted to the fact that these treatments are much less likely to cause the types of problems that standard HD does. Someone on standard HD at home may be able to deal with supplies, set-up the machine, put in the needles, monitor the treatment, take out the needles and do the clean-up. But as a care partner, you'd need to stay nearby *during the whole treatment*. You could be in a nearby room, but would have to be able to come running if the person on dialysis has a painful cramp or passes out—and then know what to do to help. In short, to do standard HD, you need to learn to be a dialysis technician. Being a tech can be a very rewarding role. Some people truly enjoy it and do it for years, or even decades. The clinic that trains you will tell you how to set-up respite treatments if you need a break or have somewhere else you need to be.

- **Short Daily HD** – Most short daily HD programs require someone to have a care partner. But, for short daily HD, you should not be the one who learns to become a tech. During training (which may take from 2–6 weeks), *the person on dialysis* should learn to be his or her own tech. You can be an extra pair of hands, help with trouble shooting, and take on any role you work out for supplies, set-up, and/or clean-up. Major problems during short daily HD treatments are *very rare*. You *can* be somewhere else in the house—folding laundry, working in a home office, etc. during short daily HD, with a cell phone or bell as a signal if you're needed. Or, a number of people use short daily HD time to play cards, watch movies, or invite friends over. Needing to be there for five or six 2.5–4 hour short daily HD treatments does take a good chunk of time out of your week—up to 24 hours or so. Talk about a schedule ahead of time or at the start of each week to be sure it will work for both of you. Yes, short daily HD treatments can be flexible—but it's not fair for someone on short daily HD to just inform you of when you'll be needed from day to day. You're a care partner, not a servant! The more the person on short daily HD can do, the easier it is to find and train someone else to help out if you need a night out or you travel for work. Standard in-center HD is always an option for respite as well.

- **Nocturnal Home HD** – Most home nocturnal HD programs also require a care partner—though we know of people who dialyze safely at home without one. Nocturnal HD is a very safe, gentle treatment. Training for nocturnal HD tends to take longer than short daily HD training—about 4–8 weeks. Just how long the training will take will depend on how long it takes to learn the equipment and the steps and feel confident. As with short daily HD, the person doing nocturnal HD should take on the bulk of the tasks and be the "tech." As a care partner, once training is done, nocturnal HD will take far less time out of your week than short daily HD. Even if you do all of the set-up and clean-up (which we don't suggest), it's about 45 minutes per treatment, or up to 4.5 hours per week. Alarms going off at night can interrupt your sleep. And supply orders and delivery, if you help with them, add a few hours per month, too.

Coping with HD Needles

If you are thinking of helping someone to do home HD, it is best if the person who does HD puts in the needles. He or she is the only person who can feel *both* ends of the needle. In some cases, this won't work, due to vision problems, hands that don't work well, or an access that is impossible to reach. (Notice that we didn't say anything about being right or left handed. People do seem to be able to figure out how to use their non-dominant hand to put in HD needles, even if they can't write or brush their hair with it.) If the person on HD *can't* put his or her needles in, this task may fall to you.

There is no doubt that the idea of putting HD needles into *anyone*—let alone someone you care about—can be terrifying. The needles are large (and they may loom even larger in your mind). Putting them in can hurt, even if it's a brief hurt, and will need to happen whether you do it or not. If you have needle fear yourself, and many do, even getting up the courage to look at the needles can be a big step.

We do hope you'll think about it, though. Because **the fewer people who put needles into an access, the longer it will last**. Staff in a clinic need to move from one person to the next and the next and the next. They're in a hurry, and mistakes happen. It's not hard to learn one access and you can take as much time as you need. A healthy access lifeline means a healthier person on HD. Access infections and problems are a leading cause of death on HD. Helping someone with the needles so he or she can dialyze at home is truly a gift of a better life.

Open the Lines of Communication

Doing home dialysis of *any* type is about more than just doing the steps, keeping logs, and dealing with supplies. When you are a care partner, you also have a relationship to maintain and strengthen. Adding home dialysis into your life is like adding a new puppy or a baby to your home. Suddenly, there is a whole new list of tasks that must be done. Someone will need to put away the supplies so you can find them when you need them. Set up a machine and test all of the alarms. Fill out log sheets. Put in and tape down the needles, or connect a catheter. You get the picture.

If you live with someone else, at some point you had to figure out who pays the bills and who cleans the bathroom. Who does the laundry and who mows the lawn. Who cooks and who cleans up. Perhaps you've changed these roles over time. Switching from standard in-center HD to home offers a chance for someone to have more energy and take back some of the roles in your household that he or she may have given up. But it adds a number of new tasks, too, and you'll both need to decide who will do what.

Your home training nurse can help you make out a checklist. Talk to each other about who will do which tasks. If it doesn't work out the way you planned, try to be open to trading tasks, or taking on more yourself. How well you can work together to figure this out is a good sign of how well you'll succeed.

Give and Take

Give some thought to the give and take of the relationship itself, too. When you do nothing but give, you may risk burnout. If you're a neighbor or friend of the person on dialysis, perhaps you're helping out for money or free rent. That's a fair exchange. So is feeling that you and the person you're helping are *on the same team* to improve his or her health so you can have a better (and longer) life together. But helping with dialysis because you are in a relationship with someone who says you are "supposed to," or you are being forced into it, or made to feel guilty, is not a good sign.

When a relationship is not balanced or healthy, it can work for quite a while when you don't spend much time alone. But home dialysis means you *will* spend more time together. We hope that you and your partner respect, love, and support each other. We hope you feel you're on the same team. We hope you can talk about things that bother you without

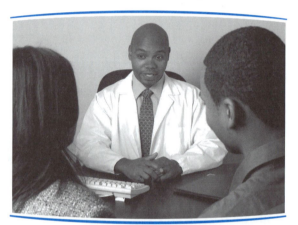

having to worry about stepping on emotional landmines—or even abuse. If you or your partner bully or scorn each other, we doubt that home dialysis will succeed for long.

Counseling can work wonders for helping you and your partner to adjust to kidney failure and take on the challenge of home treatment together. It can give you and your partner a chance to talk things through with someone who doesn't judge you, but rather helps you to find your own answers. Ask the dialysis social worker to help you and your loved one work better together. Just adjusting to the life changes caused by kidney failure can be a good reason to seek counselling. It can be the best money you ever spend.

Burnout and Respite Care

When you travel by air, a flight attendant gives a safety talk. In it, he or she will tell you that in the event that the plane descends, oxygen masks will drop down—and you need to put *your* mask on first before you help someone else. As a home HD care partner, you need to care for yourself, too.

Life happens whether or not someone you care for is on dialysis. Perhaps another family member is ill, or you have a lot of work travel, there is just simply too much on your plate—or you need to get away for a bit. Don't wait for burnout to happen! Ask for help early if you need it.

Home HD programs have respite options for those times when you need a break. Your loved one can dialyze in-center while you have some time off, either as standard treatments, in-center nocturnal, or possibly in-center self-care with a NxStage machine. Or, some people hire a nurse or tech as a helper for a few treatments if they must be away. Don't be afraid to use these options. You need to put your oxygen mask on first.

System of Dialysis Care and Medicare 101

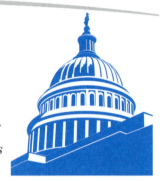

Dialysis in the U.S.—both home dialysis and standard in-center HD—is provided through clinics that are certified by Medicare or the Veteran's Administration. Also called "units," "centers," or "facilities," dialysis clinics must follow a set of Medicare rules called the *Conditions for Coverage* that were first released in 1976, and were updated in 2008.

If Medicare is your primary payer, your clinic will bill Medicare for dialysis. The clinic gets a "bundled" payment that must cover your treatments, supplies, staff time, intravenous meds, and some lab tests. The amount starts at $229.63 per treatment. This "base" payment can then be adjusted up *or* down. A "wage index" means clinics in different towns will get a different rate. And, "case-mix" adjustment means the age and health of the person getting dialysis affects the payment. During the first 4 months of treatment, Medicare pays 51% more. So, for each person, the bundled amount can vary by quite a bit. Since you will end up paying 20% of the final amount out of pocket or with another health plan, this affects you.

Each clinic must have certain staff, called the "care team," to provide care to people using home treatments and standard in-center HD:

- A medical director
- Registered nurses (at least one per shift)
- A registered renal dietitian
- A social worker with a master's degree

Clinics in every state except Montana also have dialysis techs, who provide direct care to standard in-center HD patients. Techs are required to have training plus on-the-job supervision before they can provide care by themselves. After the training, each nurse may supervise three or more techs on each shift. Each tech may care for four or more people on dialysis at a time. Each state decides how many techs and nurses must be on hand to care for people on dialysis. Medicare now requires techs to be certified. This means they have to pass an exam, and then may need to get continuing education credits each year.

There are more than 5,000 dialysis clinics in the U.S. that are certified by Medicare, and they are organized much like restaurants. About a third are either independent (think "mom and pop diner") or part of small to medium clusters of clinics with a single owner, often a doctor. A few clinics are still hospital-based, but most are free-standing. About two thirds of all U.S. clinics are owned by one of two *large dialysis organizations* or LDOs (corporate "chains," like McDonald's). See Chapter 14 for the largest dialysis companies in the U.S. right now.

Dialysis Oversight

Where you live, there may be only one clinic, or you may have many to choose from. A system of **ESRD Networks** oversees dialysis in the U.S. The Networks are Medicare contractors, and have three key jobs:

- **They collect data about each person on dialysis and send it to Medicare.** These data become the United States Renal Data System (USRDS) Annual Data Report. No names are used, but this report gives the "big picture" of dialysis care in the U.S.

- **They monitor quality in each clinic in their region.** The Networks track whether or not clinics are meeting quality benchmarks. If they are not, steps can be taken to address this.

- **They handle complaints from people on dialysis.** Each Network has a Patient Services Coordinator (PSC) and a Medical Review Board that includes some people who have kidney failure. If you have a problem that you can't work out at your clinic— or your clinic kicks you out—you can call your Network for help. In Chapter 14, you'll find the map of ESRD Networks and a chart of phone numbers for the PSCs.

Medicare 101

In the late 1960s, dialysis was experimental and in short supply. In 1972, the Medicare ESRD Program was passed, after people with kidney failure and doctors spoke and wrote to Congress. To this day, there are three ways to get Medicare:

- Be over age 65
- Be disabled and received Social Security disability checks for 24 months
- Have kidney failure

Medicare can cover U.S. citizens of *any* age who need dialysis or a kidney transplant if they qualify. To qualify, you must have enough work credits to be able to receive Social Security. About 93% of Americans qualify.

How to Qualify for Medicare

Besides needing dialysis or a kidney transplant, to get Medicare for kidney failure you need to have work credits. You get credits by earning money in each quarter of a year. Each year, the amount you must earn to get a credit goes up. In 2011, you need to earn at least $1,120 in a quarter to get a credit. You can earn up to 4 credits a year, one per quarter.

The younger you are, the fewer work credits you need to qualify for Social Security. If you're under 24, the most credits you would need are 6. If you're 24 through 30, you need more. By age 62, you need 40 credits, or a total of 10 years of work. Social Security can tell you how many credits you have and how many you need.

Haven't worked outside the home? You may still qualify for Medicare if your spouse has worked enough. Even if you're divorced or widowed, a former spouse's credits count for your Medicare if you were married for at least 10 years—and haven't remarried before age 60.

A parent's work credits can qualify a child for Medicare, too. And, in some cases, an adult child's work credits can help a dependent parent over age 65 to qualify. (NOTE: Using someone else's work credits to get Medicare does not take any credits away from their record.)

How Medicare Works

Medicare Part A (hospital care) is free if you have enough credits. There is a premium if you don't have enough credits. As long as you're on dialysis or within 36 months of a transplant, you can work and keep Part A for free. Workers with other disabilities can keep Medicare Part A for free for 8.5 years, and after that by paying for it. Or, some states will pay their premiums if they qualify for a program called "Qualified Working Disabled Individual."

Medicare Part B (medical) has a monthly premium. Parts A and B both have deductibles to pay before Medicare starts to pay. Do you have low income and few assets? You can apply for a Medicare savings program though your state's Medicaid or Medi-Cal (in California) agency to help pay your premiums. With a low enough income (up to 135% of the Federal poverty level), and few assets, your state will also help pay your Part A and B deductibles and the 20% Medicare co-pay.

Medicare Part C is known as a Medicare Advantage Plan. This type of plan covers hospital and medical expenses. If you had a Medicare Advantage Plan before your kidneys failed, you can keep it. Some Medicare Advantage special needs plans will take people whose kidneys have failed. They may pay for some things other plans will not, but may cost you more.

Medicare Part D pays for prescription drugs. Anyone who has Medicare can buy a Part D plan. There is a premium, and there are deductibles to pay. You will need to choose a plan that will pay for the drugs you take, but the plans can change. Each year, you can choose a new plan if you need to. Ask Medicare how to do this by calling 1-800-MEDICARE.

Primary and Secondary

When someone has two health plans, the plans may coordinate benefits. Medicare is **primary** if you don't have an employer group health plan. This means it pays first. When Medicare is primary, it will pay 80% of the "usual and customary" fee for dialysis. You will need to pay the other 20% by using Medicaid (if you have it), a Medigap plan if you can get one, a non-group plan, or your own funds.

If you have a group health plan through an employer, the law says *that plan is primary for the first 30 months*. It pays first—and Medicare (if you choose to take it) is **secondary**. It pays some part of the balance that your first plan doesn't cover. The 30-month "clock" starts when you become eligible for Medicare—whether you take it or not.

Here's a key question: Why pay for Medicare Part B if you have an employer group health plan? Here are three reasons:

1. When you have a primary *and* a secondary plan, you're likely to pay less out of pocket. Charges that are not paid by one plan may be paid by the other.

2. Any health care provider that "accepts assignment" agrees to take 100% of Medicare's allowed charges as payment in full. ***This means if your health plan pays at least as much as Medicare allows, your dialysis clinic can't bill you for more***. Doctors and other health care staff who accept Medicare can't charge you more, either. So, having Medicare and using health care providers that accept assignment can save you thousands of dollars more than you would pay for the Part B premiums.

3. Clinics charge private insurance companies at rates that are much closer to the true cost of care. This extra income is what keeps the whole dialysis system afloat. So, when you have an employer health plan, you are more attractive to the clinic. Your employer plan may pay for more dialysis and transplant options than Medicare.

Home Dialysis and Medicare

Medicare kicks in at different times, based on which type of treatment you choose. For standard in-center HD, Medicare will not start to pay until your third full month of treatment. This means *you* will have to pay any bills for hospitals, doctors, etc. that

Keep a Close Eye on Your Employer Group Health Plan

Do you know the dollar limit on your health plan? Many policies have a $1 million lifetime benefit. That may sound like a lot of money. But when you have one or more surgeries, perhaps some time in intensive care after a heart attack, and then you start dialysis, it can add up in a huge hurry. If you use up your lifetime benefit, it may be hard to get other health insurance.

In one recent court case, a dialysis company was billing $2,000 per dialysis treatment. At three standard HD treatments per week, this is $24,000 per month, or $288,000 per year—without drugs or any other health care. You can see that it would not take long to use up $1 million at this rate.

Be sure that your dialysis clinic is "in network" for your insurance. Getting "out of plan" or "out of network" care can mean tens of thousands of dollars in extra bills.

aren't paid by other health insurance. These charges can add up to thousands or even tens of thousands of dollars. But, you can get Medicare on the *first day* of the month you start dialysis if you start a home training program. This was done on purpose by Medicare to encourage people to do home dialysis. (NOTE: You must start to train for a home treatment before your third full month of dialysis.)

Whether you choose peritoneal dialysis (PD) or HD, you'll need surgery to create an access. If you don't have health insurance, this can cost you thousands of dollars. But when you *start* home training **before your third full month of treatment**, you may be able to get Medicare back dated so it will pay for access surgery that is done in the month you start dialysis. Table 11-1 below shows how this can work:

Table 11-1: Medicare Timeline

Dialysis Option	November Partial month of dialysis	December 1st full month	January 2nd full month	February 3rd full month
In-center HD	■ You have access surgery after the 1st of the month. ■ Your access heals and is ready to use. ■ You have your 1st treatment.	You do in-center HD all month.	You do in-center HD all month.	**Medicare does not start until the 1st of this month**
PD or Home HD	■ You have access surgery after the 1st. ■ Your access heals and is ready to use. ■ You have your 1st treatment. **Medicare starts on the 1st of this month**	You do standard HD or start PD or home HD training.	Or, you start PD or home HD training now.	You are training for PD or home HD or doing home PD or HD.

What Medicare Pays for at Home

Many people think that if they do dialysis at home, they have to buy or rent the machine. Not true! It's the job of the dialysis clinic to train you and to give you a machine and supplies. **Medicare (or your insurance) pays for the machine—you don't have to buy it**.

Medicare also pays for up to 15 days to train you for PD (most people learn how in a week or two) and up to 2 months in three 5-hour training sessions a week for home HD (25 sessions at most, but most people learn in less time).

Recliner Chairs for Home HD

If you plan to do standard or short daily home HD (treatments you would sit in a chair to do), **what Medicare pays for your dialysis treatments includes paying for your clinic to give you a basic adjustable chair (recliner)**. This item is considered "support equipment" because it is "medically necessary" for you to be able to recline in case your blood pressure drops. For this reason, a dialysis chair is listed in the Medicare Benefit Policy Manual, Chapter 11, sections 10 (D6 under Definitions) and 50.3. The chair Medicare expects the clinic to provide will not warm up, vibrate, rock, or swivel. If you want these features and are willing to pay for them, talk to your clinic when they order your chair.

We have had many complaints from people whose clinics told them they had to buy a dialysis chair themselves. If you have Medicare as your primary payer and your clinic will not give you a chair, Medicare may consider this to be fraud. Talk to your clinic, show them this page of the book, and ask them to look up the policy if you need to. If the clinic won't help, look up your ESRD Network (in Chapter 14) and call the Patient Services Coordinator, or contact your State Survey Agency. Contact information for your ESRD Network and the State Survey Agency for your area should be posted on the wall in your clinic.

If you do home HD, your clinic will supply:

- The HD machine
- An IV pole
- Water treatment equipment (if needed)
- A manual blood pressure cuff
- A stethoscope
- Enough dialyzers to do three treatments per week
- Enough blood tubing to do three treatments per week
- Dialysate and supplies to test it
- Supplies such as gloves, tape, gauze, etc.
- Chemicals to sterilize your machine (if needed)
- Saline fluid for flushing
- Dialysis needles
- Heparin to thin your blood
- Needles and syringes
- Chair

If you do PD, your clinic will supply:

- A PD cycler if you use one
- A manual blood pressure cuff
- A stethoscope
- A dialysate heater if you don't use a cycler
- An IV pole
- Dialysate fluid
- Tubing
- Supplies such as gloves, tape, gauze, etc.
- A start-up kit with a scale, thermometer, scissors, clamps, etc.
- Antibiotics for an infection
- EPO, other IV drugs, and some oral drugs

Some home HD machines require wiring or plumbing changes. Medicare will pay for minor changes to connect to water and electricity that is in your home now. Medicare will *not* pay to run new water and electricity lines to the room you want to use for treatments—but some clinics will pay for these changes if they are needed.

Medicare pays for *three* HD treatments per week. In some cases, your doctor can write a letter to Medicare and they will allow one more payment per week. This fourth payment can make it possible for a clinic to offer you daily home HD or nocturnal home HD more than three nights per week. Or, if you have an employer group health plan, it may pay for more treatments.

Minimizing your dialysis costs

There are steps you can take to pay less for dialysis:

- Ask your doctors if they accept Medicare assignment. All dialysis clinics do.
- Tell your doctor, clinic, and other healthcare providers what health coverage you have and always report any changes in coverage right away.
- Apply for Medicare and ask for it to start the first date you're eligible.
- Apply for Medicaid (Medi-Cal in California) if you have limited income and assets.
- Ask the Medicaid caseworker if you qualify for a Medicare savings program to pay premiums, deductibles, and co-pays, and apply if you do.
- Ask your state insurance department if you can get a Medigap plan and apply for one. (NOTE: You will have to pay for a Medigap plan.)
- Ask Social Security to see if you qualify for Part D "Extra Help." If you do, it can save you thousands of dollars on drugs you take at home.
- If your income is too high for Medicaid but you can't afford your premiums, ask your dialysis social worker if you can get help to pay your premiums from the American Kidney Fund.

Besides having control over your own treatment and schedule, choosing PD or home HD for your first treatment can save you thousands of dollars out-of-pocket each year for hospitals, doctors, and dialysis. Give home dialysis a try. You'll be glad you did!

Choosing a Dialysis Clinic

The most important thing for you to know about dialysis clinics is that they can differ—a *lot*. Most people choose a clinic based on where their doctor sends them, how close it is to home, or how easy it is to get to. But some clinics offer *much* higher quality care than others. Some offer only one form of treatment—while others offer several in-center and home types so you have more options. You have a right to choose your doctor and your clinic (you'll want to choose one your insurance will pay for).

Getting good quality care helps you to have the best life possible on dialysis. There are a number of different ways that quality is checked and improved in dialysis:

- **State Medicare Surveyors** inspect each clinic to ensure that they follow Medicare rules. Inspections can be done at any time if there is a complaint. If no complaints are made, clinics get surprise visits as time permits. A U.S. General Accounting Office (GAO) study in October, 2003 found that, while states are expected to survey all of their dialysis clinics within 3.5 years, only nine states met this goal. Five percent had not been seen in 9 years. The same surveyors often must visit nursing homes and other institutions, too. Since laws require nursing homes to be inspected every year, dialysis clinics are a lower priority.

- **Large dialysis organizations** track the care given in their own clinics. They do *continuous quality improvement* (CQI) projects to help all of their clinics improve their outcomes. Independent clinics may also do CQI projects to improve care. Medicare Surveyors must ask clinics about their CQI programs when they do an inspection.

- **National statistics on kidney failure**, including age, gender, and race; treatment type; cause of kidney disease; measures of quality; and much more, are collected each year. They are compiled into a resource called the *United States Renal Data System* (USRDS) Annual Report. These statistics are used to look at national and regional trends and see if care is getting better across the country. You can download the USRDS report at www.usrds.org/adr.htm.

- **The End-Stage Renal Disease (ESRD) Networks** track a set of "Clinical Performance Measures" (CPMs) of dialysis quality. They report on these in the USRDS Annual Data Report. Networks also provide some education and do CQI projects.

- **Clinical Practice Guidelines** put out by the National Kidney Foundation (NKF) address some aspects of care. The guidelines are based on medical research and the thoughts of a national expert panel. *These guidelines are a minimum.* Care that meets—*or exceeds*—KDOQI Guidelines is what you'll want to look for.

What to Look for in a Standard HD Clinic

When you do your treatments in a clinic—day or night—that clinic becomes a big part of your life. You get to know the staff and the other people on dialysis. We *strongly* urge you to visit a clinic before you decide to get treatment there. Here are some things you can look for or ask about:

- **Setting** – Does the clinic neighborhood seem safe, and if not, will a security guard be outside? Are the outside doors kept locked? Is there parking, and if so, is it free? Is the parking lot well lit and well kept? If you will need to take a bus, is there a stop nearby?

- **Clinic** – Does the clinic *look* and *smell* clean? Can you get in and out if you need to use a walker, cane, or wheelchair? Does the room temperature seem comfortable? Are there TVs for people to watch during treatment? If you speak a language other than English, or you are hearing impaired, how often will they have an interpreter to help you? How much privacy would you have?

- **Staff** – The clinic will have a "personality" that depends on who runs it and the attitudes of the people who work there. Watch how the staff talk to people on dialysis. Are they friendly and respectful? Yelling across the room to each other?

- **Rules** – When you get your treatment in a clinic, they will give you a list of their rules. Rules can differ a lot from one clinic to the next. Ask if you can have a visitor during treatment, if you can eat or drink, or if you can use a laptop or a cell phone. Be sure you can live with the rules your clinic sets, or look for one that is less restrictive.

- **Support** – How will the clinic help you learn what you need to know when you first start treatment? Do they offer a newsletter? A support group for people on dialysis or for their families? Teaching days? Videos? Look around to see if there are educational materials in the waiting room, and ask about their education program.

Look Up Your Clinic

It's always good to visit a dialysis clinic and see it for yourself. But, there are some things you can't see—like how well other people do who get their treatment from that clinic. Propublica, an independent, non-profit news source, has built a database of all of the U.S. dialysis clinics. You can see it at: http://projects.propublica.org/dialysis.

In the database, you can see which clinics are close to you, and how well they care for people on dialysis.

- **Outcomes** – How good is the care a clinic delivers? Ask what types of treatment they offer and if they plan to add any new treatments in the near future, so you have more choices. Ask the administrator or nurse manager how many hospital days people tend to have per year, and what percent of people die.

- **Emergency plan** – What will the clinic do if there is a fire? If it must close due to a flood or blizzard? Do they have a plan to deal with pandemic flu? The clinic should be able to describe what it will teach you and what you will need to do if there is an emergency when you are at treatment or between treatments. You'll need to know where to get updates in case of bad weather or other problems that could close a clinic.

Medicare suggests that you also look for the answers to questions like these:[1]

- What are the clinic hours? Do they change at the holidays?
- Does the clinic have a defibrillator in case someone has a heart problem?
- Can you talk to others who are doing dialysis at the clinic?
- What sort of education or exercise program is offered?
- Are dialyzers reused?
- What treatment shift would I get—how much choice would I have about this?
- Are numbing medications offered for needle placement?
- Will you have a choice about who puts in the neeedles?
- Will the clinic teach you how to put your own needles in if you want to learn this?

In many cases, you will have a choice of more than one clinic. If your health plan or where you live gives you only one choice and you *don't* like that choice, you may want to think about moving, choosing a home option, or working with your health plan to see if you can get another choice. Medicare has a website where you can look at the quality of a dialysis clinic: www.medicare.gov/dialysis. You may need to change doctors to go to a different clinic. If you choose to get your treatments in a clinic, the choice of clinic could have more impact on you, day by day, than your doctor. So, a change might be worth it.

For Home Dialysis, Bigger is Often Better

So, you've done your homework and want to do dialysis at home. And you've chosen the type of treatment you want to do. But *where*? If you have more than one choice of home clinic, how do you decide which will be the best fit for you? If you're looking for clinics that offer any of the types of home dialysis, visit our "Find a Clinic" database on Home Dialysis Central (www.homedialysis.org).

If you are thinking of doing PD or home HD, a key question to ask a home program is, ***"How many people are doing my treatment choice at your clinic?"*** For a home dialysis program, bigger *is* better. It may seem that a program with 2 or 3 people doing home treatments might give you lots of personal attention. But in a small program, the home training nurse—your main contact—will likely spend time in both the home and the standard HD clinic. The result: less time for you.

Successful home programs say that each full-time home training nurse can train and support about 20 people. So, a program with 20 people on peritoneal dialysis (PD) or home hemodialysis (HD) may have a nurse just for home. A program with 40 people will likely have *two* nurses—so they can take turns being on call, and can both answer questions.

Some programs have gone to a regional model instead of having lots of small programs. This means a bit more driving, but it may be better for you.

Larger programs may have other pluses, too:

- Policies that evolved through trial and error may be more user-friendly for you
- More experience with the types of challenges you might run into
- More people doing your type of treatment who may be willing to talk with you

No large program in your area?

- **Look in a wider area**. A home dialysis clinic doesn't have to be right around the corner—it can be as far away as you are willing to drive once a month for clinic visits. We know of people who even moved to another city or state to get the treatment they wanted.
- **Offer to be a peer mentor**. You can help a smaller program grow by volunteering to talk to other people who are doing standard in-center HD and might be interested in home. Ask your local paper or magazine to write a feature story about you. Talk at health fairs. Happy customers are the best salespeople for home treatments.

Look for Experienced Staff

Another key question to ask a home program is, ***"What is the home dialysis background of the training nurse(s)?"***

In the Conditions for Coverage (the Medicare rules for dialysis clinics) section 494.140(b)(2), it lists the experience a home training nurse must have:

"(2) *Self-care and home dialysis training nurse.* The nurse responsible for self-care and/or home care training must—

(i) Be a registered nurse; and

(ii) Have at least 12 months experience in providing nursing care and an additional 3 months of experience in the specific modality for which the nurse will provide self-care training."

This level of training and experience is a *minimum*. If the *only* program in your area has staff who are new to home dialysis, ask what resources they have to help them solve challenges. Or, you may find yourself doing a lot of problem solving on your own or online.

Ask *how many* people the nurse has trained. A nurse who has trained only a handful of people may not be as helpful as someone who has trained a dozen or more. Ask to meet the person who will do your training, too—not just the program director. Be sure that you can work with the nurse who will train you.

How Are People on Home Dialysis at This Clinic Doing?

Sure, home treatments are work friendly. They may be easier to fit into your schedule. They can help you regain control of your life. But the reality is, you do end up with set-up and clean-up, supplies to order and track, treatment logs to keep and send in, and a fair amount of work to do.

The real benefit of home treatments is that you can feel better, have a more normal diet, stay out of the hospital more—and even live longer. So, ask ***"What are the clinical outcomes of people who are doing the type of treatment I want?"***

If you plan to do PD, ask about infections. Good clinics may have just one infection per several *years* of PD. This means they're doing a great job of training—and of motivating people to do their PD with care.

If you plan to do home HD, ask the program what outcomes they are tracking and how people are doing. If they can answer you, it's a good sign that they are paying attention. The data they collect can also help to prove that home HD is a better, safer treatment option than standard in-center HD.

Will You Choose Me?

Programs differ in their beliefs about who is best suited to do a home treatment. This means *"How will you decide if I can do home treatment at your clinic?"* may get a different answer, based on where you go.

We encourage clinics to use our **Method to Assess Treatment Choices for Home Dialysis (MATCH-D)** tool.[2] This tool helps clinics assess people for home treatments and overcome any challenges they might have. It can be downloaded at www.homedialysis.org/match-d

We believe the best predictor of home dialysis success is *how motivated you are to do your treatments at home*. A clinic that would turn you down because you are a minority, older, a single parent, can't hear well, etc. may not be one you'd want to go to anyway. If a clinic turns you down for home treatment and you *know* you can do it, look for another clinic.

Do-it-*Yourself* Hemodialysis

A home program's philosophy of care has a lot to do with how much *you*—vs. a partner—will do on home HD. Research has found that when someone on dialysis does more (and the partner, if there is one, does less), success is more likely.[3-5] So, ask the program, *"How much of my treatment do you expect me to do, vs. a partner?"*

A clinic that says, "we'll teach *you* to do as much as you can" has your best interests at heart. A clinic that trains your partner to be your tech—while you sit as "the patient"—may be setting you *both* up to fail.

Many partners find putting in dialysis needles to be *very* stressful. Placing your own needles may make you more likely to succeed in the long-term. If you *truly* can't do it (i.e., you don't have the use of one hand), be sure to thank your partner for making it possible for you to be home. Often.

A few programs don't require a partner—but may require a Lifeline® button device that can call 911 or someone who can reach you quickly if you hit a snag.

If you are quite ill when you start home HD, you may not feel well enough at first to take on a lot of your care. When you start to feel better, take some of the burden off of your partner by doing what you can by yourself. And be sure to say "thank you" for what your partner does for you. Showing appreciation can mean a lot.

Talk To Me About Training

How long will it take me to get a training slot? If you have a good job with a health plan and want to keep it, this is a key question. You may be better off seeking out a clinic that can get you in sooner rather than waiting months and risking losing your job. (You can do standard in-center HD while you wait, but may not feel as well—or the time slot may not fit with your job.)

What will my training schedule be? Ask to see the training plan and find out what a typical day will be like. What will you learn when? How long might it take? Can it be done around your work day?

Will I and my care partner (if I have one) train alone, or with others? Some clinics train 2–4 people (and partners if they have them) in small groups. This can be a way to shorten waiting lists and create a built-in support group for people on dialysis and partners. If your learning styles are very different, having someone else there could push you faster than you'd like, or slow you down. Whether you prefer one-on-one or group training is a personal decision, but it's something you'll want to ask about.

Home Sweet Home Visits

"Will you do a home visit when I start doing my treatments by myself?" Most programs will do a home visit before you start home training, to see how your home can be set-up to make things easier on you. A home visit can help you figure out the best place to set-up your machine or store supplies—or how to have pets and do home treatment safely. But the first treatment at home on your own is still stressful. Your nurse may visit for your first treatment to ease your transition. Whether you do PD or home HD, a home visit can help you start off on the right foot.

Even after you get started, some programs will do a home visit to be sure that you have what you need, and to help you troubleshoot if you run into a problem.

Don't Be a Dropout!

What percentage of your people go back to standard HD? Most people who do treatments at home feel much better. But treatment at home may not involve just you—it can throw a wrench into your home life if you are not ready for it. Each year, as many as 30–40% of people who start home treatments decide to quit—most in the stressful first 3 months.

Some programs do a better job than others of supporting both people on dialysis and partners (when present)—and they have very low dropout rates.

The difference? They make sure that you know exactly what to expect, and plan who will do which tasks. They take their time during training so you feel confident that you can handle things—and even bring you back in for a refresher if you need it. They call you to see how you're doing and if you have questions you haven't gotten a chance to ask. They focus on making your life work for you (not on making you fit into their structure).

Conclusion

Home dialysis can improve your life—and choosing a good clinic can make your home treatment experience better.

How to Protect Yourself in the Hospital

The Hippocratic Oath that all doctors must take says, in part, "above all, do no harm." Doctors and hospitals do not set out to harm anyone, but mistakes do happen. People are human, and that includes people in healthcare. Each year in the U.S., the Institute of Medicine says that nearly 100,000 people die due to medical errors. Countless more are injured, some permanently. Many of these errors occur in hospitals. The single most important thing you can do is *be active in your care*. Know your treatment, your meds, and ask questions.

Hospital nurses are busy, and you may have to wait to get what you need. While in the hospital it is best if you can have someone with you who knows your wishes. You may need more than one person to do this. The more severe your problem is, the more vital it is to have someone who is there just for you.

Your advocate can be your eyes, ears, and legs. To reduce drug errors, an FDA rule requires hospitals to have bar code systems that match your ID bracelet with your drugs before you get them. Your advocate can double check that this is done. He or she can watch you for changes, and do other small helping tasks. Unless your advocate has had hospital training, he or she should not help you get out of bed without a trained staff person to help. You don't want to risk a fall that could injure you both.

Ask Questions and Know Your Rights

Learn your options if you need a procedure. Is there more than one way to achieve the same result? How many times has the doctor done the procedure? Practice makes perfect: it is safer to go to someone who has done the procedure you need *at least 25 times during training*.[1] It's okay to ask about this. If the doctor has not (or has done so only a few times), do you have a second choice of doctor or hospital?

What kinds of anesthesia can you have? For a short procedure, are you better off with local or spinal anesthesia instead of general? Often, you'll have a choice. Before you leave post-op after a procedure, be sure your pain is controlled—or you'll be playing "catch-up" to try to get on top of the pain. Ask for more meds if you need them.

Do you go to a teaching hospital? If so, you always have the right to refuse to permit medical students to be present. If you can plan your stay, avoid late nights or weekends—very little happens then.

Across the U.S., residency programs for doctors in training start on July 1. This is a good reason *not* to have elective surgery in July. If you *must* be in a hospital in July, ask about the training of each doctor who sees you. Insist that the *staff doctor* do your procedure—not a doctor in training. You can add this to your surgical consent form.

You can ask to read your chart each day, to be sure that your blood tests look good and your recovery is going well. Ask for a copy of your hospital's Patient Bill of Rights. If you do run into a snag, each hospital has a Patient Representative who can help resolve disputes. Ask the nurse to call this person for you if you need to.

In-hospital Dialysis

In most hospitals, dialysis is done by acute care nurses at the bedside or in a small unit. You may have one nurse who gets to know you very well and is there for each treatment. But, even acute care nurses may not know about PD, daily, or nocturnal home hemodialysis (HD). And the floor nurses may not know about dialysis at all. This is where mistakes can be made.

Are you on PD? Call your PD nurse before you enter the hospital, or as soon as you can once you're there. It is safest if you can do your own exchanges if you feel up to it. If not, *only* permit staff who are trained in PD, do your exchanges, so you avoid infection. Floor staff need to know that **your PD catheter is for dialysis only**—it is not a way to give drugs or nutrition. You can get peritonitis if your catheter is misused. Ask for a sign above your bed, and have someone write this with a surgical marker on your belly if you will not be conscious at any time during your stay.

When peritonitis brings you to the hospital, you may need to do HD until you heal. If you don't have an HD access, a temporary HD catheter will be placed. When your stay is for a hernia repair or other problem, you may be able to do low-volume, recumbent-only (LVRO) PD (while lying flat) and avoid an HD catheter.

When you do any form of HD and are in the hospital, you need to protect your access—and your access arm. Do not let anyone take your blood pressure on that arm or draw blood from an access site. It's a good idea to post a sign on the wall by the bed to alert hospital staff about your HD access.

If you do daily or nocturnal HD, you may be able to keep doing this in the hospital. If not, you will need to adjust your diet for standard HD. **Failing to limit potassium when you switch to standard HD can be fatal.** Choose foods that are on your diet. If you did not choose a meal, don't assume that your tray has the right foods—mistakes happen. *Look* at what you get. Ask before you eat or drink something you're not sure of.

Ask about each drug you are given *before* you take it—including IV drugs. Is it the right drug for you? The correct dose? Is the drug safe for people with kidney failure? Has your kidney doctor been consulted? Are your fluid levels being watched, since you may not make much (or any) urine? If you have diabetes, your blood sugar control can be thrown off by the change in routine, illness, or stress. Check your sugars and be sure your insulin or oral drugs are adjusted, too.

Prevent Infection

With so many sick people in one place, hospitals are hotbeds of infection. *Any surface in a hospital can harbor harmful bacteria—wash your hands often.* You can help protect yourself if you:[2]

- ☐ Check that staff wash their hands or use alcohol-based cleanser before they touch you. Gloves protect *them*—not you. The gloves may be dirty.
- ☐ With kidney failure, your immune system may not work as well. A private room can help you avoid infection.
- ☐ Ask your visitors to wash their hands.
- ☐ Be sure stethoscopes are wiped with an alcohol pad before use.
- ☐ Choose a surgeon with a low infection rate if you need surgery.
- ☐ If surgery is planned ahead, shower each day with 4% chlorhexidine soap (e.g., Hibiclens) for 3 to 5 days. A drugstore can order this for you without a prescription.
- ☐ Are you a carrier of *staphylococcus aureus*? Ask for a simple swab of your nose. If you are a carrier, your risk of infection is greater. Your care team can take extra steps to protect you from infection.
- ☐ Do you smoke? Quitting before surgery improves blood flow and helps speed healing.
- ☐ Ask about getting an antibiotic one hour before surgery. This helps reduce the risk of infection.
- ☐ Using a warming blanket during surgery can help you fight infection afterward.
- ☐ If hair must be removed from a surgical site, a clipper is safer than shaving, which leaves tiny nicks in your skin.
- ☐ Refuse to allow extra people (like medical students) in the operating room—each brings bacteria in.
- ☐ Note when your IV is placed—it should be changed every 3 to 4 days.

Pack a Hospital Kit

Any time you go to the ER, you may be admitted. Pack a small bag with a folder of key papers and comfort items—and you'll have what you need. Include:

- ☐ An up-to-date list of drugs you take, the dose, and how often you take each one (*don't* bring your own drugs)
- ☐ Your medical history, including your dialysis prescription
- ☐ Contact information for your doctor and dialysis clinic
- ☐ All of your health insurance and/or Medicare cards
- ☐ A list of phone numbers of loved ones
- ☐ A hair brush, toothbrush, toothpaste
- ☐ Hand sanitizer to keep by your bedside
- ☐ Underwear, warm socks, and a pair of slippers with rubber soles
- ☐ A black-out sleep mask and ear plugs to help you sleep
- ☐ Your own pillow or neck pillow, if you prefer a special kind
- ☐ Books, magazines, or puzzles in case you need something to do
- ☐ A comfortable change of clothes to wear home

The hospital will provide gowns, robes, and towels—you don't need to bring these. Most hospitals have a TV set for each bed, with many channels that may include radio. Bring a cell phone and charger if you have one. You may want to bring a laptop—if you can lock it to a table to secure it. Like jewelry, computers may be stolen.

Tip: Leave your watch, jewelry, and valuables home, so you don't have to worry about losing them. Don't bring credit cards or large amounts of cash.

Conclusion

You can't always avoid a hospital stay, but you can take steps to protect your comfort and safety while you're there.

Resources

Websites

The Internet offers a vast array of information. To search for information, go to www.google.com and put the term you are looking for into the search box. If you don't have a computer or know how to use one, ask a family member, neighbor, or friend for help, or go to the library and the librarian can help you. Look for sites that have HON (Health on the Net) certification to be sure you can trust the information. Don't trust testimonials or sure cures—sadly, there are many scams on the Internet, and there is no cure for chronic kidney disease.

Below, we list some websites that have helpful information for people with kidney disease. There are many more.

■ **Home Dialysis Central** – a Medical Education Institute, Inc. website to raise awareness and use of PD and home HD. Talk to others on home dialysis in our forums, find a clinic in our database, read stories, see equipment, and much more. Sign up for a free monthly e-newsletter. www.homedialysis.org.

■ **Kidney School** – a Medical Education Institute website to help people learn how to self-manage stage 3–5 chronic kidney disease. Kidney School is free, and offers 16 self-paced modules online, as downloadable PDFs, or as audio books, at www.kidneyschool.org. Topics include:

Module 1 - Kidneys: How They Work, How They Fail, What You Can Do
Module 2 - Treatment Options for Kidney Failure
Module 3 - Working with Your Health Care Team
Module 4 - Following Your Treatment Plan
Module 5 - Coping with Kidney Disease
Module 6 - Anemia and Kidney Disease
Module 7 - Understanding Kidney Lab Tests
Module 8 - Vascular Access: A Lifeline for Dialysis
Module 9 - Nutrition and Fluids for People on Dialysis
Module 10 - Getting Adequate Dialysis
Module 11 - Sexuality and Fertility
Module 12 - Staying Active with Kidney Disease
Module 13 - Heart Health and Blood Pressure
Module 14 - Patient Rights and Responsibilities
Module 15 - Alternative Treatments
Module 16 - Long-term Effects of Dialysis

- **Life Options** – a Medical Education Institute, Inc. website dedicated to helping people live long and live well with kidney disease, with a wealth of free info for patients and professionals at www.lifeoptions.org.

- **Nocturnal Dialysis** – Dr. Agar has built a comprehensive site with information about nocturnal hemodialysis in Austrialia, at www.nocturnaldialysis.org.

- **DaVita** – One of the largest U.S. dialysis providers has built a website with education, videos, recipes, tools, and much more. Check out the Diet Helper, Treatment Evaluator, and Food Analyzer. www.davita.com.

- **Dialysis Facility Compare** is Medicare's site to compare the quality of dialysis clinics. The site has been criticized because the data tend to be a year or two old, and are pretty general. But it's a good place to start. www.medicare.gov/dialysis.

- **Dialysis-Support** is an email support listserv with members at all stages of kidney disease who help and support each other. An email listserv is a group of people who share something in common. When an email from one person is sent to the list, each member receives it. This can mean getting a lot of email. For this reason, listservs can be set for individual emails, or a single digest of all of the emails sent in one day. To join this group, visit http://groups.yahoo.com online. In the "Find a Yahoo Group" box, put Dialysis-Support. Then click *Join this group*.

- **Dialysis from the Sharp End of the Needle** – a blog started by long term dialyzor and global traveler, Bill Peckham, to track industry news and trends in advocacy, reimbursement, payment, and the provision of dialysis. www.billpeckham.com.

- **Fistula First** – if you can have one, an arteriovenous fistula is the best access for dialysis. This website has resources to help you learn about the steps involved in getting a fistula. www.fistulafirst.org/patients.aspx.

- **Fresenius** – The largest U.S. dialysis provider's website will help you find a nephrologist or a clinic, analyze your food, understand treatment options, sign up for classes, and much more. www.ultracare-dialysis.com.

- **Hemodoc** – physician Peter Laird started dialysis in 2007 and quickly switched to home treatments. His blog site has his observations about dialysis, and lots of good information. www.hemodoc.com.

- **Medicare.gov** – Medicare pays for most dialysis in the U.S. On this site, find reams of helpful information about Medicare, drug plans, and much more. Put "Dialysis" into the search box to find Medicare booklets for you. www.medicare.gov.

- **Propublica** – this independent, non-profit newsroom has built a database of U.S. dialysis clinics, and you can look up your clinic and see how it compares to others. http://projects.propublica.org/dialysis.

Voluntary Kidney Organizations

Support and information are key to living well with kidney disease, and an array of organizations offer both. These include:

- **The American Association of Kidney Patients** is a membership organization with a magazine, free materials, and an annual patient meeting: www.aakp.org.

- **The American Kidney Fund** offers direct financial help to patients, and much more: www.akfinc.org.

- **Dialysis Patient Citizens**, which has more than 22,000 members, is working to improve quality of life for all people on dialysis. www.dialysispatients.org.

- **The Kidney Transplant/Dialysis Association (KT/DA)** provides financial aid, information, and emotional support to kidney patients and families: www.ktda.org.

- **The National Kidney Foundation** has a patient and family council, and local chapters in many states: www.kidney.org.

- **The Oxalosis and Hyperoxaluria Foundation (OHF)** is a gateway to information about these kidney-stone producing conditions. Learn all about it at www.ohf.org/index.html.

- **The Renal Support Network** helps link kidney patients together through "Bridge" groups for education, support, and advocacy: www.renalnetwork.org.

Care Partner Resources

- ***When the Man You Love is Ill: Doing Your Best for Your Partner Without Losing Yourself.*** By Dorree Lynn & Florence Isaacs. 2007. ISBN#: 1569242852. (This book is not just for partners of men.)

- **Family Caregiver Alliance**
  FCA seeks to improve quality of life for caregivers through education, services, research, and advocacy. FCA's National Center on Caregiving offers information on current social, public policy and caregiving issues, and offers help to develop public and private programs for caregivers.
  180 Montgomery Street, Suite 1100
  San Francisco, CA 94104
  415-434-3388 or 800-445-8106
  www.caregiver.org

- **National Family Caregivers Association (NFCA)**
  NCFA educates, supports, and advocates for the more than 50 million Americans who care for loved ones with a chronic illness, disability, or frailty. NFCA reaches out to address the common needs and concerns of all family caregivers.
  10400 Connecticut Avenue, Suite 500
  Kensington, MD 20895-3944
  301-942-6430 or 800-896-3650
  www.thefamilycaregiver.org

■ **Johnson & Johnson/Rosalynn Carter Institute Caregivers Program**

The mission of J&J/RCI is to enhance the quality of life, quality of care, knowledge, and understanding of family caregivers. We recognize that the future of our nation's health care system rests on the shoulders of the family caregivers, who are major providers of long-term care. Caregiver needs must be addressed in a timely, caring, and competent way to ensure the health and well-being of both the caregiver and the person(s) they are caring for.

www.rosalynncarter.org

■ **National Alliance for Caregiving (NAC)**

Established in 1996, The NAC is a nonprofit coalition of national groups that focus on family caregiving.

4720 Montgomery Lane, 5th Floor
Bethesda, MD 20814

www.caregiving.org

■ **Share the Care**

Share the care has resources to help you put together a team to care for someone who is very ill.

www.sharethecare.org

■ *Today's Caregiver*

Today's Caregiver magazine includes up-to-the-minute advice and interviews with celebrity caregivers such as Dana Reeve, former First Lady Rosalynn Carter and Debbie Reynolds; information on caregiver.com includes topic-specific channels, free weekly email newsletters, and chat rooms.

www.caregiver.com

Dialysis Cookbooks, Nutrition, and Exercise Guides

If you do standard HD, the easiest way to adapt to the new diet limits is to make changes to recipes you already enjoy. But cookbooks can also give you new ideas. Here are some we found on Amazon.com that you may be able to order at your local bookstore (use the ISBN number). Some are older and may be hard to find:

■ *Bowes and Church's Food Values of Portions Commonly Used* – by Jean A.T. Pennington and Judith S. Spungen. 2009. ISBN# 9780781781343.

■ *Cleveland Clinic Foundation Creative Cooking for Renal Diets* – by Cleveland Clinic Foundation. 1985. ISBN# 9780941511889.

■ *Cleveland Clinic Foundation Creative Cooking for Renal Diabetic Diets* – by Cleveland Clinic Foundation. 1985. ISBN# 9780941511896.

■ *Cooking for David, a Culinary Dialysis Cookbook* – by Sara Colman and Dorothy Gordon. 2000. ISBN# 0970161700.

■ *Exercise, a Guide for People on Dialysis* – by Patricia Painter, PhD. Free download from: www.lifeoptions.org/catalog/pdfs/booklets/exercise.pdf.

■ *The Renal Patient's Guide to Good Eating: A Cookbook for Patients by a Patient* – by Judith A. Curtis and Thomas Batis. 1989. ISBN# 0398073996.

■ *Silver Spoons: Hemodialysis Cookbook* – by Dave Capper. 2010. ISBN# 1449977529.

Dialysis Equipment Makers

If you have questions or problems with home dialysis equipment, the manufacturers can be a good source of information to help you.

- Baxter – PD equipment; has a new home HD machine in the pipeline. Call toll-free: 800-422-9837, www.baxter.com.

- Fresenius – PD equipment; 2008K@home HD machine; has a new home HD machine in the pipeline. Call toll-free: 866-4DIALYSIS, www.fmcna.com.

- NxStage – System One home HD machine and PureFlow device. Call toll-free: 866-697-8243, www.nxstage.com.

Largest U.S. Dialysis Providers[1]

Company	# Clinics	# People Cared for on Dialysis
Fresenius Medical Care North America 866-434-2597 | www.ultracare-dialysis.com	1688	123,363
DaVita Inc. 800-244-0680 | www.davita.com	1450	114,500
Dialysis Clinic Inc.* 615-327-3061 | www.dciinc.org	210	12,980
Renal Advantage Inc. † 615-661-1100 | www.renaladvantage.com	137	10,664
DSI Renal Inc.** 615-777-8200 | www.dsi-corp.com	113	7,692
American Renal Associates 877-997-3625 | www.americanrenal.com	80	5,000
Liberty Dialysis LLC † 206-236-5001 | www.libertydialysis.com	96	4,940
Satellite Healthcare Inc. § 650-404-3600 | www.satellitehealth.com	44	4,009
Innovative Dialysis Systems 562-495-8075 | www.idsdialysis.com	44	3,385
U.S. Renal Care Inc. 214-736-2700 | www.usrenalcare.com	61	3,196

DCI is the only company on this list that is a non-profit

** *DSI has been bought by DaVita*

† *Liberty and Renal Advantage have merged together for purchasing purposes, and were purchased by Fresenius.*

§ *Satellite's WellBound division focuses on home dialysis and has more than 1,000 people dialyzing at home*

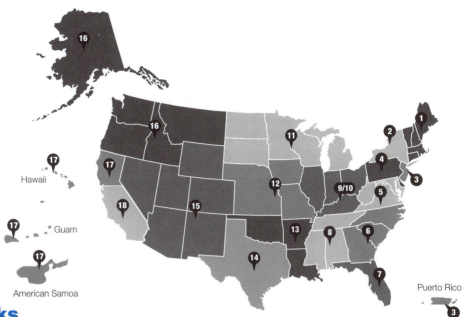

ESRD Networks

ESRD Network Number & Name	States Covered	Phone Number
1. ESRD Network of New England	Connecticut, Maine, Massachusetts, New Hampshire, Rhode Island, Vermont	1-866-286-3773
2. IPRO ESRD Network of New York	New York	1-800-238-3773
3. Transatlantic Renal Council	New Jersey, Puerto Rico, Virgin Islands	1-888-877-8400
4. ESRD Network 4, Inc.	Delaware, Pennsylvania	1-800-548-9205
5. Mid-Atlantic Renal Coalition	Maryland, Virginia, DC, West Virginia	1-866-651-6272
6. Southeastern Kidney Council	Georgia, North Carolina, South Carolina	1-800-524-7139
7. FMQAI: The Florida ESRD Network	Florida	1-800-826-3773
8. Network 8, Inc.	Alabama, Mississippi, Tennessee	1-877-936-9260
9/10. The Renal Network, Inc.	Indiana, Kentucky, Ohio, Illinois	1-800-456-6919
11. Network of the Upper Midwest, Inc.	Michigan, Minnesota, North Dakota, South Dakota, Wisconsin	1-800-973-3773
12. Heartland Kidney Network	Iowa, Kansas, Missouri, Nebraska	1-800-444-9965
13. ESRD Network 13	Arkansas, Louisiana, Oklahoma	1-800-472-8664
14. ESRD Network of Texas, Inc.	Texas	1-877-886-4435
15. Intermountain ESRD Network	Arizona, Colorado, Nevada, New Mexico, Utah, Wyoming	1-800-783-8818
16. Northwest Renal Network	Alaska, Idaho, Montana, Oregon, Washington	1-800-262-1514
17. Western Pacific Renal Network, LLC	American Samoa, Guam, Hawaii, Mariana Islands, Northern California	1-800-232-3773
18. Southern California Renal Disease Council	Southern California	1-800-637-4767

Glossary

Abbreviations

APD	automated peritoneal dialysis, done with a cycler
AVF	arteriovenous fistula
B2M	beta-2 microglobulin; a middle molecule waste (see Amyloidosis)
Ca	calcium
Ca x P	calcium phosphorus product; a measure of risk for extraskeletal calcification
CAPD	continuous ambulatory peritoneal dialysis
CCPD	continuous cycling peritoneal dialysis
CFU	colony-forming units; a measure of bacteria in dialysis water
CHF	congestive heart failure
CKD	chronic kidney disease
CMS	Centers for Medicare and Medicaid; Medicare
CRP	C-reactive protein; a measure of inflammation
EDW	estimated dry weight
eGFR	estimated glomerular filtration rate; a measure of kidney function
EPO	erythropoietin; a hormone that tells your bone marrow to make red blood cells
ESAs	erythropoiesis stimulating agents; medications that tell your bone marrow to make red blood cells
ESRD	end-stage renal disease; a legal term for kidney failure
EU	endotoxin units; a measure of bacterial toxins in dialysis water
GFR	glomerular filtration rate
HD	hemodialysis
HeRO®	"hemodialysis reliable outflow;" a type of dialysis access that links a graft to a central vein in the chest
HIPAA	Health Insurance Portability and Accountability Act – law that ensures privacy of medical records
IJ	internal jugular
LVH	left ventricular hypertrophy; overgrowth and weakness in the heart's main pumping chamber
Kt/V	a measure of how much urea is removed during dialysis
PD	peritoneal dialysis
pH	measure of acidity
PKD	polycystic kidney disease
PTH	parathyroid hormone
RBCs	red blood cells; erythrocytes
RLS	restless legs syndrome
URR	urea reduction ratio; a formula to measure how much urea is removed during dialysis

Terms

Access – a way to reach the blood to do dialysis. PD uses an abdominal or presternal catheter for access. HD access is through a central venous catheter, graft, or, the "gold standard," an arteriovenous fistula.

Adequacy – the minimum amount of dialysis needed to maintain life.

Advance directive – a "living will," health care proxy, and/or power of attorney for health-care matters. An advance directive is a way to share your health care wishes in case there is a time when you cannot speak for yourself.

Albumin – a type of protein that is measured in your blood. Levels below 4.0 g/dL suggest a risk of malnutrition.

Alum – an aluminium compound added to clarify city water. Can be harmful to people on dialysis.

Amyloidosis – build up of a waxy protein, called amyloid, in soft tissues or joints, when levels of B2M in the blood are too high.

Anemia – shortage of oxygen-carrying red blood cells.

Aneurysm – a weak, thin spot in a blood vessel wall that can balloon outward and possibly burst.

Arteriovenous fistula – a type of hemodialysis access in which a surgeon sews an artery to a vein under the skin of an arm. Blood flow from the artery enlarges the vein so it can be used for dialysis.

Aseptic – sterile; germ-free.

Back filtration – movement of germs through a filter into the body.

Biocompatible – like the human body.

Buttonhole technique – placing dialysis needles in the exact same spots at the exact same angle until a "tunnel" tract forms, much like a pierced earring hole, to guide the needles into a fistula with less pain and less risk of aneurysms. Care must be taken to remove the scabs after each treatment using aseptic technique to avoid infection.

Calciphylaxis – a rare condition in which crystals of bone form in small blood vessels, cutting off blood supply and creating a risk of gangrene, limb loss, and death.

Catheter – a tube. A catheter can be used as an access for PD or for HD. HD catheters are best for short-term use only, as the risk of infection is very high.

Congestive heart failure – a condition in which a weakened heart cannot pump enough blood, so some blood backs up into the lungs and tissues. Excess blood volume (in kidney failure) can cause or worsen this problem.

Creatinine – a waste produced each time you move your muscles that is removed by healthy kidneys. Rising levels in the blood are a possible sign of kidney disease.

Depression – a common mood disorder that may include feelings of sadness, loss of interest or pleasure, feelings of guilt or low self-worth, sleep problems, low energy levels, and poor mental focus. Depression can be treated.

Dialysate – a precise mix of water and chemicals into which wastes flow during dialysis.

Dialysis – the process of cleaning wastes and excess water out of the blood using osmosis and diffusion.

Dialyzer – artificial kidney.

Diffusion – the process by which dissolved wastes in your blood shift from one fluid space to another until the levels are equal in all three spaces.

Dry weight – your weight without any extra water in your blood.

Electrolytes – dissolved salts that carry an electrical charge.

Endotoxin – toxic parts of bacteria cell walls that are freed when the bacteria die, and can contaminate dialysis water and cause fever and chills.

Erythropoietin – a hormone made by the kidneys that tells the bone marrow to make red blood cells.

Euvolemia – the same amount of fluid comes into the body and leaves it.

Extracellular – outside and between the cells; fluid that bathe and nourish the cells.

Extraskeletal calcification – bone that forms in the soft tissues, joints, or blood vessels.

Fistula – see arteriovenous fistula.

Fluid spaces – the three places in the body where fluid can go: inside cells, outside cells, and in the bloodstream.

Glomerular filtration rate – percent of kidney function.

Glomerulus – a tangled capillary blood vessel ball that forms part of a nephron.

Gradient – a difference in the level of solutes between two or more fluid spaces in the body used in dialysis to remove wastes.

Graft – a dialysis access in which an artery is connected to a vein under the skin of your arm, using a piece of man-made vein.

Hemodialysis – a type of dialysis where the blood is passed through a filter to remove wastes and excess fluid.

Heparin – a blood thinning drug.

High flux – flux means flow. A high flux dialyzer has larger pores (holes) that let more and larger wastes flow through.

Homeostasis – a constant environment inside your body.

Icodextrin – a PD fluid that is based on a starch, rather than dextrose (sugar). It is less likely to cause scarring of the peritoneal membrane, but costs more.

Infiltration – placement of a dialysis needle through the back wall of a fistula or graft, causing bleeding into the tissues, bruising, and pain.

Internal jugular – vein in the neck that is the preferred spot for a central venous hemodialysis catheter, if one is needed.

Interstitial – outside and between the cells; fluid that bathe and nourish the cells. Extracellular.

Intracellular – inside the cells.

Malnutrition – too few nutrients to support health.

Medicare – a U.S. government health insurance program that is open to citizens who are over age 65, disabled, or have kidney failure and who qualify based on their work records.

Membrane – thin layer of tissue that forms a barrier. In dialysis, blood and dialysate interact through a membrane.

Middle molecule – a waste with a molecular weight between 500 and 12,000 daltons. Middle molecules are linked with long-term complications of standard HD, such as joint damage.

Modality – mode or type of treatment.

Nephrogenic systemic fibrosis – a syndrome that has been linked to use of gadolinum contrast dye for MRI tests, causes thick skin, stiff joints, lung fibrosis, and heart damage, and can be fatal.

Nephrology – the study of kidneys and kidney disease.

Nephrologist – doctor who specializes in treating kidney disease.

Nephron – filtering unit of the kidney made up of a glomerulus and a tubule.

Neuropathy – nerve damage.

Nocturnal hemodialysis – overnight dialysis treatments, done at home 3–6 nights per week, or in a clinic 3 nights per week. The slower treatments are more gentle on the heart, remove far more wastes and water than standard treatments, and take less time out of the day.

Omentum – a "curtain" of tissue inside the abdomen that can get in the way of peritoneal dialysis, and is therefore sometimes removed when a PD catheter is placed.

Osmosis – the process by which shifting of fluid across a semipermeable membrane occurs until levels are equal on both sides of the membrane. Salt or sugar can create a gradient that forces fluid to shift.

Pathogen – harmful germ.

Peritoneal dialysis – a treatment for kidney failure that uses the lining of the inside of the abdomen as a filter to clean the blood. A surgeon places a catheter through the wall of the belly or chest, which is used to fill the abdomen with sterile fluid. Wastes and water from the blood flow into the fluid, which is then discarded and replaced with fresh.

Peritoneum – single layer of cells lining the inside of the abdomen.

Phosphorus – a mineral that, together with calcium, forms most of the bones and teeth, and is found in the blood in small amounts. Phosphorus is found in most foods and can build up to levels in kidney failure that lead to itching and bone problems.

Physiologic – like the human body.

Presternal catheter – a type of PD catheter that is placed through the wall of the chest and reaches down into the abdomen. The chest wall is thinner and cleaner than the wall of the abdomen. A presternal catheter can also allow tub bathing, though not swimming.

Pruritus – itching.

Pseudoporphyria – a skin disorder found in people on standard HD. The skin may develop purple spots, tear easily, and heal slowly.

Pyrogenic reaction – fever response to a toxin from dialysis water.

Reframing – looking at the same thing in a different way.

Restless legs syndrome – a sleep disorder in which a "creepy crawly" sensation occurs that is improved only by movement.

Self-management – deciding what to eat and drink, managing symptoms, taking pre-scribed drugs, following a treatment plan, and advocating for yourself.

Short daily hemodialysis – a type of treatment for kidney failure in which 2–3 hour treatments are done 5–6 days per week, using a specially designed small machine. Doing treatments more than 3 days per week removes more water, more gently, reduces heart damage, lowers blood pressure, and helps people feel better physically.

Solutes – dissolved wastes that must be removed from the blood.

Ultrafiltration – removal of water from the blood during dialysis.

Uremia – a group of symptoms that occur when wastes build up in the blood due to kidney failure.

References

Chapter 1

1. National Kidney Association. Chronic Kidney Disease accessed July 20, 2011 from http://www.kidney.org/kidneydisease/ckd/index.cfm

2. Blagg CR. The early history of dialysis for chronic renal failure in the United States: a view from Seattle. *Am J Kidney Dis.* 2007 49(3):482-96

3. U.S. Renal Data System, 2011 USRDS Annual Data Report: Atlas of Chronic Kidney Disease and End-Stage Renal Disease in the United States, National Institutes of Health, National Institute of Diabetes and Digestive and Kidney Diseases, Bethesda, MD, 2011.

4. USRDS 1997 Annual Data Report, USRDS Dialysis Morbidity and Mortality (Wave 2), p. 53

5. Campbell A. Strategies for improving dialysis decision making. *Perit Dial Int.* 1991 11:173-178

6. Stack AG, Martin DR. Association of patient autonomy with increased transplantation and survival among new dialysis patients in the United States. *Am J Kidney Dis.* 2005 45(4):730-42

7. Merighi JR, Schatell DR, Bragg-Gresham JL, et al. Insights into nephrologist training, clinical practice, and dialysis choice. *Hemodialysis Int*, in press, January 2012

Chapter 2

1. Lopes AA, Bragg J, Young E, et al. Dialysis Outcomes and Practice Patterns Study (DOPPS). Depression as a predictor of mortality and hospitalization among hemodialysis patients in the United States and Europe. *Kidney Int.* 2002 62(1):199-207

2. Andresen EM, Malmgren JA, Carter WB, et al. Screening for Depression in Well Older Adults: Evaluation of a Short Form of the CES-D. *Am J Prev Med.* 1994 10(2):77-84

3. Miller WC, Anton HA, et al. Measurement properties of the CESD scale among individuals with spinal cord injury. *Spinal Cord.* 2008 46:287-292

4. Radloff LS. The CES-D scale: A self-report depression scale for research in the general population. *Appl Psychol Meas.* 1977 1:385-401

5. Radloff LS, Locke BZ. The community mental health assessment survey and CES-D Scale. In *Community surveys of psychiatric disorders*, MM Weissman, JK Myers, and CE Ross (Eds). 1986 Rutgers University Press: New Brunswick, NJ. p. 177-187

6. Swenson SL, Rose M, Vittinghoff E, et al. The influence of depressive symptoms on clinician-patient communication among patients with type 2 diabetes. *Med Care.* 2008 46(3):257-65

7. Lindquist H. The old man: My death with dignity. Accessed July 20, 2011 from http://maplewood.blogs.nytimes.com/2009/07/02/the-old-man-my-death-with-dignity/

Chapter 3

1. Ehler JT. Accessed July 20, 2011 from http://www.foodreference.com/html/fwatercontent.html

2. Yavuz A, Tetta C, Ersoy FF, et al. Uremic toxins: a new focus on an old subject. *Semin Dial.* 2005 18(3):203-11

Chapter 4

1. Kjellstrand CM, Evans RL, Petersen RJ, et al. The "unphysiology" of dialysis: a major cause of dialysis side effects? *Kidney Int.* 1975 Suppl 2:30-4.

2. Narita I, Iguchi S, Omori K, et al. Uremic pruritus in chronic hemodialysis patients. *J Nephrol.* 2008 21(2):161-5

3. Lin HH, Liu YL, Liu JH, et al. Uremic pruritus, cytokines, and polymethylmethacrylate artificial kidney. *Artif Organs.* 2008 32(6):468-72

4. Akhyani M, Ganji MR, Samadi N, et al. Pruritus in hemodialysis patients. *BMC Dermatology.* 2005 24;5:7

5. Noordzij M, Boeschoten EW, Bos WJ, et al; for the NECOSAD Study Group. Disturbed mineral metabolism is associated with muscle and skin complaints in a prospective cohort of dialysis patients. *Nephrol Dial Transplant.* 2007 22(10):2944-9

6. Wikstrom B. Itchy skin—a clinical problem for hemodialysis patients. *Nephrol Dial Transplant.* 2007 22 Supple 5:v3-7

7. Pifer TB, McCullough KP, Port FK, et al. Mortality risk in hemodialysis patients and changes in nutritional indicators: DOPPS. *Kidney Int.* 2002 62(6):2238-45

8. Chung SH, Lindholm B, Lee HB. Is malnutrition an independent predictor of mortality in peritoneal dialysis patients? *Nephrol Dial Transplant.* 2003 18(10):2134-40

9. Locatelli F, Buoncristiani U, Canaud B, et al. Dialysis dose and frequency. *Nephrol Dial Transplant.* 2005 20(2):285-96

10. Sarris E, Tsele E, Bagiatoudi G, et al. Diffuse alopecia in a hemodialysis patient caused by low-molecular weight heparin, tinzaperin. *Am J Kidney Dis.* 2003 41(5):E15

11. Apsner R, Horl WH, Sunder-Plassmann G. Dalteparin-induced alopecia in hemodialysis patients: reversal by regional citrate anticoagulation. *Blood.* 2001 1;97(9):2914-5

12. National Kidney Foundation. KDOQI Clinical Practice Guidelines and Clinical Practice Recommendations for Anemia in Chronic Kidney Disease. *Am J Kidney Dis.* 47:S1-S146, 2006 (suppl 3). Accessed July 20, 2011 from http://www.kidney.org/professionals/KDOQI/guidelines_anemia/cpr12.htm accessed July 20, 2011

13. Dandona P, Dhindsa S, Chandel A, et al. Hypogonadatrophic hypogonadism in men with type 2 diabetes. *Postgrad Med.* 2009 121(3):45-51

14. Malavige LS, Levy JC. Erectile dysfunction in diabetes mellitus. *J Sex Med.* 2009 6(5):1232-47

15. Karacan I, Salis PJ, Hirshkowitz M, et al. Erectile dysfunction in hypertensive men: sleep-related erections, penile blood flow and musculovascular events. *J Urol.* 1989 142(1):56-61

16. Veronelli A, Mauri C, Zecchini B, et al. Sexual dysfunction is frequent in premenopausal women with diabetes, obesity, and hypothyroidism, and correlates with markers of increased cardiovascular risk. A preliminary report. *J Sex Med.* 2009 6(6):1561-8

17. Enzlin P, Rosen R, Wiegel M, et al.; DCCT/EDIC Research Group. Sexual dysfunction in women with type 1 diabetes: long-term findings from the DCCT/EDIC study cohort. *Diabetes Care.* 2009 32(5):780-5

18. Fatemi SS, Taghavi SM. Evaluation of sexual function in women with type 2 diabetes mellitus. *Diab Vasc Dis Res.* 2009 6(1):38-9

19. Doumas M, Tsiodras S, Tsakiris A, et al. Female sexual dysfunction in essential hypertension: a common problem being uncovered. *J Hypertens.* 2006 24(12):2387-92

20. Francis ME, Kusek JW, Nyberg LM, et al. The contribution of common medical conditions and drug exposures to erectile dysfunction in adult males. *J Urol.* 2007 178(2):591-6

21. Araujo AB, Travison TG, Ganz PA, et al. Erectile dysfunction and mortality. *J Sex Med.* 2009 6(9):2445-54

22. Khatana SA, Taviera TH, Miner MM, et al. Does cardiovascular risk reduction alleviate erectile dysfunction in men with type II diabetes mellitus? *Int J Impot Res.* 2008 20(5):501-6

23. Lu CC, Jiann BP, Sun CC, et al. Association of glycemic control with risk of erectile dysfunction in men with type 2 diabetes. *J Sex Med.* 2009 6(6):1719-28

24. Zofkova I, Bubenicek P, Sotorni'k I. [Hypogonadism, a serious complication of chronic renal insufficiency] Article in Czech. *Vnitr Lek.* 2007 53(6):709-14

25. Messina LE, Claro JA, Nardozza A, et al. Erectile dysfunction in patients with chronic renal failure. *Int Braz J Urol.* 2007 33(5):673-8

26. Kettas E, Cayan F, Akbay E, et al. Sexual dysfunction and associated risk factors in women with end-stage renal disease. *J Sex Med.* 2008 5(4):872-7

27. Lessan-Pezeshki M, Ghazizadeh S. Sexual and reproductive function in end-stage renal disease and effect of kidney transplantation. *Asian J Androl.* 2008 10(3):441-6

28. Williams SW, Tell GS, Zheng B, et al. Correlates of sleep behavior among hemodialysis patients. The kidney outcomes prediction and evaluation (KOPE) study. *Am J Nephrol.* 2002 22(1):18-28

29. Han SY, Yoon JW, Jo SK, et al. Insomnia in diabetic hemodialysis patients. Prevalence and risk factors by a multicenter study. *Nephron.* 2002 92(1):127-32

30. Parker KP, Kutner NG, Bliwise DL, et al. Nocturnal sleep, daytime sleepiness, and quality of life in stable patients on hemodialysis. *Health Qual Life Outcomes.* 2003 1:68

31. Unruh ML, Hartunian MG, Chapman MM, et al. Sleep quality and clinical correlates in patients on maintenance dialysis. *Clin Nephrol.* 2003 59(4):280-8

32. Sanner BM, Tepel M, Esser M, et al. Sleep-related breathing disorders impair quality of life in haemodialysis recipients. *Nephrol Dial Transplant.* 2002 17(7):1260-5

33. Mucsi I, Molnar MZ, Rethelyi J, et al. Sleep disorders and illness intrusiveness in patients on chronic dialysis. *Nephrol Dial Transplant.* 2004 19(7):1815-22

34. Rijsmn RM, de Weerd AW, Stam CJ, et al. Periodic limb movement disorder and restless leg syndrome in dialysis patients. *Nephrology (Carlton).* 2004 9(6):353-61

35. Azar SA, Hatefi R, Talebi M. Evaluation of the effect of renal transplantation in treatment of restless legs syndrome. *Transplant Proc.* 2007 39(4):1132-3

36. Sabbatini M, Crispo A, Pisani A, et al. Sleep quality in renal transplant patients: a never investigated problem. *Nephrol Dial Transplant.* 2005 20(1):194-8

37. Sato M, Morita H, Ema H, et al. Effect of different dialyzer membranes on cutaneous microcirculation during hemodialysis. *Clin Nephrol.* 2006 66(6):426-32

38. Masmoudi A, Ben Hmida M, Mseddi M, et al. [Cutaneous manifestation of chronic hemodialysis. Prospective study of 363 cases] Article in French. *Presse Med.* 2006 35(3 Pt 1):399-406

39. Koszo F, Foldes M, Morvay M, et al. [Chronic hemodialysis-related porphyria/pseudoporphyria]. Article in Hungarian. *Orv Hetil.* 1994 135(39):2131-6

40. Cooke NS, McKenna K. A case of haemodialysis-associated pseudoporphyria successfully treated with oral N-acetylcysteine. *Clin Exp Dermatol.* 2007 32(1):64-6

41. Massone C, Ambros-Rudolph CM, Di Stefani A, et al. Successful outcome of haemodialysis-induced pseudoporphyria after short-term oral N-acetylcysteine and switch to high-flux technique dialysis. *Acta Derm Venereol.* 2006 86(6):538-40

42. Vadoud-Seyedi J, de Dobbeleer G, Simonart T. Treatment of haemodialysis-associated pseudoporphyria with N-acetylcysteine: report of two cases. *Br J Dermatol.* 2000 142(3):580-1

43. Agarwal R, Brunelli SM, Williams K, et al. Gadolinium-based contrast agents and nephrogenic systemic fibrosis: a systematic review and meta-analysis. *Nephrol Dial Transplant.* 2009 24(3):856-63. Comment in *Nephrol Dial Transplant.* 2009 24(7):2293; author reply 2293-4

44. Nainani N, Panesar M. Nephrogenic systemic fibrosis. *Am J Nephrol.* 2009 29(1):1-9

45. Panesar M, Banerjee S, Barone GW. Clinical improvement of nephrogenic systemic fibrosis after kidney transplantation. *Clin Transplant.* 2008 22(6):803-8

46. Kay J, High WA. Imatinib myselate treatment of nephrogenic systemic fibrosis. *Arthritis Rheum.* 2008 58(8):2543-8. Comment in *Arthritis Rheum.* 2008 58(8):2219-24

47. Mathur K, Morris S, Deighan C, et al. Extracorporeal photopheresis improves nephrogenic fibrosing dermapathy/nephrogenic systemic fibrosis: three case reports and review of literature. *J Clin Apher.* 2008 23(4):144-50

48. Piccoli GB, Fenoglio R, Colla L, et al. Cholesterol crystal embolism syndrome in dialysis patients: an emerging clinical diagnosis? *Blood Purif.* 2006 24(5-6):433-8

49. Harvey JC. Cholesterol crystal microembolization: a cause of the restless leg syndrome. *South Med J.* 1976 69(3):269-72

50. Matuszkiewicz-Rowinska J, Sko'rzewska K, Radowicki S, et al. Endometrial morphology and pituitary-gonadal axis dysfunction in women of reproductive age undergoing chronic haemodialysis—a multicentre study. *Nephrol Dial Transplant.* 2004 19(8):2074-7

51. Vidaeff AC, Yeomans ER, Ramin SM. Pregnancy in women with renal disease. Part 1: general principles. *Am J Perinatol.* 2008 25(7):385-97

52. Hou S. Historical perspective of pregnancy in chronic kidney diease. *Adv Chronic Kidney Dis.* 2007 14(2):116-8

53. Krishnan AV, Kiernan MC. Uremic neuropathy: clinical features and new pathophysiological insights. *Muscle Nerve.* 2007 35(3):273-90.

54. Ly J, Chan CT. Impact of augmenting dialysis frequency and duration on cardiovascular function. *ASAIO J.* 2006 52(6):e11-4

55. Krishnan AV, Phoon RK, Pussell BA, et al. Altered motor nerve excitability in end-stage kidney disease. *Brain.* 2005 128(Pt 9):2164-74

56. Krishnan AV, Phoon RK, Pussell BA, et al. Sensory nerve excitability and neuropathy in end stage kidney disease. *J Neurol Neurosurg Psychiatry.* 2006 77(4):548-51.

57. Espinoza M, Aguilera A, Auxiliadora Bajo M, et al. Tumor necrosis factor alpha as a uremic toxin: correlation with neuropathy, left ventricular hypertrophy, anemia, and hypertriglyceridemia in peritoneal dialysis patients. *Adv Perit Dial.* 1999 15:82-6

58. Clayton PT. B6-responsive disorders: a model of vitamin dependency. *J Inherit Metab Dis.* 2006 29(2-3):317-26

59. Moriwaki K, Kanno Y, Nakamoto H, et al. Vitamin B6 deficiency in elderly patients on chronic peritoneal dialysis. *Adv Perit Dial.* 2000 16:308-12.

60. Okada H, Moriwaki K, Kanno Y, et al. Vitamin B6 supplementation can improve peripheral polyneuropathy in patients with chronic renal failure on high-flux haemodialysis and human recombinant erythropoietin. *Nephrol Dial Transplant.* 2000 15(9):1410-3.

61. Sprenger KB, Bundschu D, Lewis K, et al. Improvement of uremic neuropathy and hypogeusia by dialysate zinc supplementation: a double-blind study. *Kidney Int.* Suppl. 1983 16:S315-8.

62. Morten IJ, Gosal WS, Radford SE, et al. Investigation into the role of macrophages in the formation and degradation of beta2-microglobulin amyloid fibrils. *J Biol Chem.* 2007 282(40):29691-700

63. Traut M, Haufe CC, Eismann U, et al. Increased binding of beta-2-microglobulin to blood cells in dialysis patients treated with high-flux dialyzers compared to low flux membranes contributed to reduced beta-2-microglobulin concentrations. Results of a cross-over study. *Blood Purif.* 2007 25(5-6):432-40

64. Menaa C, Esser E, Sprague SM. Beta2-microglobulin stimulates osteoclast formation. *Kidney Int.* 2008 73(11):1275-81

65. Okuno S, Ishimura E, Kohno K, et al. Serum {beta}2-microglobin level is a significant predictor of mortality in maintenance hemodialysis patients. *Nephrol Dial Transplant.* 2009 24(2):571-7

66. Lehmann G, Ott U, Kaemmerer D, et al. Bone histomorphology and biochemical markers of bone turnover in patients with chronic kidney disease stages 3-5. *Clin Nephrol.* 2008 70(4):296-305

67. Seyahi N, Apaydin S, Sariyar M, et al. Intracranial calcification and tumoural calcinosis during vitamin D therapy. *Nephrology (Carlton).* 2004 9(2):89-93

68. Seyahi N, Altiparmak MR, Kahveci A, et al. Association of conjunctival and corneal calcification with vascular calcification in dialysis patients. *Am J Kidney Dis.* 2005 45(3):550-6

69. Tristano AG. Metastatic calcification of the hand in a patient undergoing hemodialysis. *Am J Med.* 2004 116(8):572-3

70. Kim SJ, Goldstein M, Szabo T, et al. Resolution of massive uremic tumoral calcinosis with nocturnal home hemodialysis. *Am J Kidney Dis.* 2003 41(3):E12

71. Wang SX, Li H. Salmon calcitonin in prevention of osteoporosis in maintenance hemodialysis patients. *Chin Med J (Engl).* 2008 121(14)1280-4

72. Moe SM, O'Neill KD, Reslerova M, et al. Natural history of vascular calcification in dialysis and transplant patients. *Nephrol Dial Transplant.* 2004 19:2337-2383

73. Chertow GM, Raggi P, Chasen-Taber S, et al. Determinants of progressive vascular calcification in haemodialysis patients. *Nephrol Dial Transplant.* 2004 19(6):1489-96

74. Reslerova M, Moe SM. Vascular calcification in dialysis patients: pathogenesis and consequences. *Am J Kidney Dis.* 2003 41(3 Suppl 1):S96-9

75. Suki WN, Dialysis Clinical Outcomes Revisited Investigators. Effects of sevelamer and calcium-based phosphate binders on mortality in hemodialysis patients: results of a randomized clinical trial. *J Renal Nutr.* 2008 18(1):91-8

76. Pierratos A, Ouwendyk M, Francoeur R, et al. Nocturnal hemodialysis: three-year experience. *J Am Soc Nephrol.* 1998 9(5):859-68. Comment in *J Am Soc Nephrol.* 1998 9(5):899-900

77. Van Eps CL, Jeffries JK, Anderson JA, et al. Mineral metabolism, bone histomorphometry and vascular calcification in alternate night nocturnal hemodialysis. *Nephrology (Carlton).* 2007 12(3):224-33

78. Badve SV, Zimmerman DL, Knoll GA, et al. Peritoneal phosphate clearance is influenced by peritoneal dialysis modality, independent of peritoneal transport characteristics. *Clin J Am Soc Nephrol.* 2008 3:1711-17

79. Chacon G, Nguyen T, Khan A, et al. Warfarin-induced skin necrosis mimicking calciphylaxis: a case report and review of the literature. *J Drugs Dermatol.* 2010 859-63

80. Hayden MR, Goldsmith D, Sowers JR, et al. Calciphylaxis: calcific uremic arteriolopathy and the emerging role of sodium thiosulfate. *Int Urol Nephrol.* 2008 40(2):443-51

81. Kyritsis I, Gombou A, Griveas I, et al. Combination of sodium thiosulfate, cinacalcet, and paricalcitol in the treatment of calciphylaxis with hyperparathyroidism. *Int J Artif Organs.* 2008 31(8):742-4

82. Raymond CB, Wazny LD. Sodium thiosulfate, bisphosphonates, and cinacalcet for treatment of calciphylaxis. *Am J Health Syst Pharm.* 2008 65(15):1419-29

83. Pasch A, Schaffner T, Huynh-Do U, et al. Sodium thiosulfate prevents vascular calcification in uremic rats. *Kidney Int.* 2008 74(11):1444-53. Comment in *Kidney Int.* 2008 74(11):1376-8

84. National Kidney Foundation. KDOQI Clinical Practice Guidelines for Bone metabolism and Disease in Chronic Kidney Disease. *Am J Kidney Dis.* 2003 42(suppl 3):S1-S202. Accessed July 20, 2011 from http://www.kidney.org/professionals/kdoqi/guidelines_bone/Guide6.htm

85. Paoletti E, Specchia C, Di Maio G, et al. The worsening of left ventricular hypertrophy is the strongest predictor of sudden cardiac death in haemodialysis patients: a 10 year survey. *Nephrol Dial Transplant.* 2004 19(7):1829-34

86. Stack AG, Saran R. Clinical correlates and mortality impact of left ventricular hypertrophy among new ESRD patients in the United States. *Am J Kidney Dis.* 2002 40(6):1202-10

87. Kutlay S, Dincer I, Sengul S, et al. The long-term behavior and predictors of left ventricular hypertrophy in hemodialysis patients. *Am J Kidney Dis.* 2006 47(3):485-92

88. Paoletti E, Bellino D, Cassottana P, et al. Left ventricular hypertrophy in nondiabetic predialysis CKD. *Am J Kidney Dis.* 2005 46(2):320-7 Comment in: *Am J Kidney Dis.* 2005 46(6):1148; author reply 1148-9

89. Miyazato J, Horio T, Takiuchi S, et al. Left ventricular diastolic dysfunction in patients with chronic renal failure: impact of diabetes mellitus. *Diabet Med.* 2005 22(6):730-6

90. Koc M, Toprak A, Tezcan H, et al. Uncontrolled hypertension due to volume overload contributes to higher left ventricular mass index in CAPD patients. *Nephrol Dial Transplant.* 2002 17(9):1661-6

91. Asci G, Ozkahya M, Duman S, et al. Volume control associated with better cardiac function in long-term peritoneal dialysis patients. *Perit Dial Int.* 2006 26(1):85-8. Comment in: *Perit Dial Int.* 2006 26(1):49-52

92. Weinreich T, De los Rios T, Gauly A, et al. Effects of an increase in time vs. frequency on cardiovascular parameters in chronic hemodialysis patients. *Clin Nephrol.* 2006 66(6):433-9

93. Fagugli RM, Reboldi G, Quintaliani G, et al. Short daily hemodialysis: blood pressure control and left ventricular mass reduction in hypertensive hemodialysis patients. *Am J Kidney Dis.* 2001 38(2):371-6

94. Chan C, Floras JS, Miller JA, et al. Improvement in ejection fraction by nocturnal haemodialysis in end-stage renal failure patients with coexisting heart failure. *Nephrol Dial Transplant.* 2002 17(8):1518-21

95. Chan CT, Jain V, Picton P, et al. Nocturnal hemodialysis increases arterial baroreflex sensitivity and compliance and normalizes blood pressure of hypertensive patients with end-stage renal disease. *Kidney Int.* 2005 68(1):338-44

96. Chan CT, Floras JS, Miller JA, et al. Regression of left ventricular hypertrophy after conversion to nocturnal hemodialysis. *Kidney Int.* 2002 61(6):2235-9

97. Schatell D, Ellstrom-Calder A, Alt PS, et al. Survey of CKD patients reveals significang taps in knowledge about kidney disease. Part 1. *Nephrol News Issues.* 2003 17(5):23-6

98. Schatell D, Ellstrom-Calder A, Alt PS, et al. Survey of CKD patients reveals significang taps in knowledge about kidney disease. Part 2. *Nephrol News Issues.* 2003 17(6):17-9

99. Korevaar JC, Jansen MA, Dekker FW, et al, Netherlands Cooperative Study on the Adequacy of Dialysis Study Group. When to initiate dialysis: effect of proposed US guidelines on survival. *Lancet.* 2001 358(9287)1046-50

100. Korevaar JC, Jansen MA, Dekker FW, et al; NECOSAD Study Group. Evaluation of DOQI guidelines: early start of dialysis treatment is not associated with better health-related quality of life. *Am J Kidney Dis.* 2002 39(1):108-15

101. Cooper BA, Branley P, Bulfone L, et al; IDEAL Study. A randomized, controlled trial of early versus late initiation of dialysis. *N Engl J Med.* 2010 363(7):609-19

102. Thilly N, Boini S, Soudant M, et al. Outcomes of patients with delayed dialysis initiation: Results from the AVENIR study. *Am J Nephrol.* 2011 33(1):76-83

103. Evans M, Tettamanti G, Nyrén O, et al. No survival benefit from early-start dialysis in a population-based, inception cohort study of Swedish patients with chronic kidney disease. *J Intern Med.* 2011 269(3):289-98

104. Rosansky SJ, Eggers P, Jackson K, et al. Early start of hemodialysis may be harmful. *Arch Intern Med.* 2011 171(5):396-403

Chapter 5

1. Porazko T, Kuzniar J, Kusztal M, et al. IL-18 is involved in vascular injury in end-stage renal disease patients. *Nephrol Dial Transplant.* 2009 24(2):589-96

2. Eleftheriades T, Kartsios C, Antoniadi G, et al. The impact of chronic inflammation on bone turnover in hemodialysis patients. *Ren Fail.* 2008 30(4):431-7

3. Bradbury BD, Critchlow CW, Weir MR, et al. Impact of elevated C-reactive protein levels on erythropoiesis-stimulating agent (ESA) dose and responsiveness in hemodialysis patients. *Nephrol Dial Transplant.* 2009 24(3):919-25

4. Tonbul HZ, Demir M, Altintepe L, et al. Malnutrition-inflammation-atherosclerosis (MIA) syndrome components in hemodialysis and peritoneal dialysis patients. *Ren Fail.* 2006 28(4):287-94

5. Sato M, Morita H, Ema H, et al. Effect of different dialyzer membranes on cutaneous microcirculation during hemodialysis. *Clin Nephrol.* 2006 66(6):426-32

6. Cruz DN, De Cal M, Garzotto F, et al. Effect of vitamin E-coated membranes on anemia in patients with chronic kidney disease: an Italian multicenter study. *Int J Artif Organs.* 2008 31(6):545-52

7. Qian J, Yu Z, Dai H, et al. The study of IL-1 beta, TNF-alpha, IL-6 gene expression and plasma levels on hemodialysis before and after dialyzer reuse. *Chin Med J (Engl).* 1997 110(8):508-11

8. Muller TF, Seitz M, Eckle L, et al. Biocompatibility differences with respect to the dialyzer sterilization method. *Nephron.* 1998 78(2):139-142

9. De Cal M, Cazzavillian S, Rassu M, et al. Residual of bacterial DNA in hemodialyzers: the proof of subclinical infection sustaining chronic inflammation. *Int J Artif Organs.* 2008 31(5):395-404

10. Schwenger V. GDP and AGE receptors: mechanisms of peritoneal damage. *Contrib Nephrol.* 2006 150:77-83

11. Fusshoeller A. Histomorphological and functional changes of the peritoneal membrane during long-term peritoneal dialysis. *Pediatr Nephrol.* 2008 23(1):19-25

12. Lee YK, Lee JY, Kim JS, et al. The breakdown of preformed peritoneal advanced glycation end products by intraperitoneal alagebrium. *J Korean Med Sci.* 2009 24 Suppl:S189-94

13. Water for Hemodialysis. Association for the Advancement of Medical Instrumentation (AAMI). ANSI/AAMI RD52:2004. Approved August 9, 2004.

14. Arizono K, Nomura K, Motoyama T, et al. Use of ultrapure dialysate in reduction of chronic inflammation during hemodialysis. *Blood Purif.* 2004; 22 Suppl 2:26-9

15. Furuya R, Kumagai H, Takahashi M, et al. Ultrapure dialysate reduces plasma levels of beta(2)-microglobulin and pentosidine in hemodialysis patients. *Blood Purif.* 2005 23(4):311-16

16. Hsu PY, Lin CL, Yu CC, et al. Ultrapure dialysate improves iron utilization and erythropoietin response in chronic hemodialysis patients—a prospective cross-over study. *J Nephrol.* 2004 17(5):693-700

17. Lederer SR, Schiffl H. Ultrapure dialysis fluid lowers the cardiovascular morbidity in patients on maintenance hemodialysis by reducing continuous microinflammation. *Nephron.* 2002 91(3):452-5

18. Ash SR, Daugirdas JT. Peritoneal Access Devices. In *Handbook of Dialysis*, Third Edition, John T. Daugirdas, Peter G. Blake, Todd. S. Ing. Lippincott Williams & Wilkins, Philadelphia, 2001

19. Dasgupta MK. Moncrief-Popovich catheter and implantation technique: the AV fistula of peritoneal dialysis. *Adv Ren Replace Ther.* 2002 9(2):116-24

20. Twardowski ZJ, Prowant BF, Nichols WK, et al. Six-year experience with Swan neck presternal peritoneal dialysis catheter. *Perit Dial Int.* 1998 18(6):598-602

21. Tacconelli E, Carmeli Y, Aizer A, et al. Mupirocin prophylaxis to prevent Staphylococcus aureus infection in patients undergoing dialysis: a meta-analysis. *Clin Infect Dis.* 2003 37(12):1629-38

22. Wasse H, Speckman RA, McClellan WM. Arteriovenous fistula use is associated with lower cardiovascular mortality compared with catheter use among ESRD patients. *Semin Dial.* 2008 21(5):483-9

23. Asif A, Ravani P, Roy-Chaudhury P, et al. Vascular mapping techniques: advantages and disadvantages. *J Nephrol.* 2007 20(3):299-303

24. Goodkin DA, Pisoni RL, Locatelli F, et al. Hemodialysis vascular access training and practices are key to improved access outcomes. *Am J Kidney Dis.* 2010 56(6):1032-42

25. Hamilton JG. Needle phobia: A neglected diagnosis. *J Fam Practice.* 41(2):169-75, 1995. Full text article available free on-line at:
http://www.findarticles.com/p/articles/mi_m0689/is_n2_v41/ai_17276569 Accessed July 20, 2011

26. Oswalt RM, Napoliello M. Motivations of blood donors and nondonors. *J Applied Psychol.* 1974 59:122-24

27. McLaughlin K, Manns B, Mortis G, et al. Why patients with ESRD do not select self-care dialysis as a treatment option. *Am J Kidney Dis.* 2003 41(2):380-85

28. Peterson AL, Isler WC. Applied tension treatment of vasovagal syncope during pregnancy. *Military Med.* 2004 169(9):751-3. Full text article available free on-line at:
http://www.findarticles.com/p/articles/mi_qa3912/is_200409/ai_n9432776 Accessed July 20, 2011

29. Dhingra RK, Young EW, Hulbert-Shearon TE, et al. Type of vascular access and mortality in U.S. hemodialysis patients. *Kidney Int.* 2001 60:1443-1451

30. Lewis C. Let's empower patients with the choice of self-cannulation! *Nephrol Nurs J.* 2005 32(2):225

31. Twardowski Z, Kubara H. Different sites versus constant sites of needle insertion into arteriovenous fistula for treatment by repeated dialysis. *Dial Transplant.* 1979 8:978-80

32. Kronung G: Plastic deformation of Cimino fistula by repeated puncture. *Dial Transplant.* 1984 13(10): 635-638

33. Van Eps CL, Jones M, Ng T, et al. The impact of extended-hours home hemodialysis and buttonhole cannulation technique on hospitalization rates for septic events related to dialysis access. *Hemodial Int.* 2010 14(4):451-63

34. Schild AF, Perez E, Gillaspie E, et al. Arteriovenous fistulae vs. arteriovenous grafts: a retrospective review of 1,700 consecutive vascular access cases. *J Vasc Access.* 2008 9(4):231-5

35. Morsy MA, Khan A, Chemia ES. Prosthetic axillary-axillary arteriovenous straight access (necklace graft) for difficult hemodialysis patients: a prospective single-center experience. *J Vasc Surg.* 2008 48(5):1251-54

36. Katzman HE, McLafferty RB, Ross JR, et al. Initial experience and outcome of a new hemodialysis access device for catheter-dependent patients. *J Vasc Surg.* 2009 50(3):600-7

37. Nassar GM. Long-term performance of the hemodialysis reliable outfloe (HeRO) device: the 56-month follow-up of the first clinical trial patient. *Semin Dial.* 2010 23(2):229-32

Chapter 6

1. Bleyer AJ, Russell GB, Satko SG. Sudden and cardiac death rates in hemodialysis patients. *Kidney Int.* 1999 55(4):1553-9

2. Steering Committee for ESRD: State of the Art and Charting the Challenges for the Future; April 23-26, 2009. Letter dated June 5, 2009. Accessed July 21, 2011 at
http://www.renalweb.org/documents/ESRD_Conf_Boston_Letter.htm

3. Lockridge RS, Moran J. Short daily hemodialysis and nocturnal hemodialysis at home: practical considerations. *Semin Dial.* 2008 20(1):49-53

4. Sandroni S, Sherockman T, Hays-Leight K. Catastrophic haemorrhage from venous needle dislodgement during hemodialysis: continued risk of avoidable death and progress toward a solution. Presented at *ASN/Renal Week*, Philadelphia, Nov 2008.

5. Saner E, Nitsch D, Descoeudres C, et al. Outcome of home haemodialysis patients: a case-cohort study. *Nephrol Dial Transplant.* 2005 20(3):604-10. Comment in *Nephrol Dial Transplant.* 2005 20(8):1766; author reply 1767. *Nephrol Dial Transplant.* 2005 20(6):1272; author reply 1272

6. Moist LM, Bragg-Gresham JL, Pisoni RL, et al. Travel time to dialysis as a predictor of health-related quality of life, adherence, and mortality: the Dialysis Outcomes and Practice Patterns Study. *Am J Kidney Dis.* 2008 51(4):641-50

7. Lindsay RM, Heidenheim PA, Nesrallah G, et al. Daily Hemodialysis Study Group London Health Sciences Center. Minutes to recovery after a hemodialysis session: a simple health-related quality of life question that is reliable, valid, and sensitive to change. *Clin J Am Soc Nephrol.* 2006 1(5):952-9

8. Chesterton LJ, Selby NM, Burton JO, et al. Cool dialysate reduces asymptomatic intradialytic hypotension and increases baroreflex variability. *Hemodial Int.* 2009 13(2):189-96

9. Saran R, Bragg-Gresham JL, Levin NW, et al. Longer treatment times and slower ultrafiltration in hemodialysis: associations with reduced mortality in the DOPPS. *Kidney Int.* 2006 69(7):1222-8

10. Ball L, Hossli S, Lee E, et al. Module 6 of the *Core Curriculum for the Dialysis Technician*; Hemodialysis procedures and complications. Third Edition. ©2006 Amgen Inc. Developed by the Medical Education Institute, Inc. with support from Amgen Inc. Accessed on July 21, 2011 at http://www.meiresearch.org.

11. Young EW, Held PJ, Port FK. Nonadherence in hemodialysis: assocations with mortality, hospitalization, and practice patterns in the DOPPS. *Kidney Int.* 2003 64(1):254-62

12. Sherman RA, Mehta O. Dietary phosphorus restriction in dialysis patients: potential impact of processed meat, poultry, and fish products as protein sources. *Am J Kidney Dis.* 2009 54(1):18-23

13. Chiu YW, Teitelbaum I, Misra M, et al. Pill burden, adherence, hyperphosphatemia, and quality of life in maintenance dialysis patients. *Clin J Am Soc Nephrol.* 2009 4(6):1089-96

14. DeOreo PB. Hemodialysis patient-assess functional health status predicts continued survival, hospitalization, and dialysis-attendance compliance. *Am J Kidney Dis.* 1997 30:204-212

15. Lowrie EG, Curtin RB, LePain N, et al. Medical Outcomes Study Short Form-36: A consistent and powerful predictor of morbidity and mortality in dialysis patients. *Am J Kidney Dis.* 2003 41:1286-1291

16. Mapes DL, Lopes AA, Satayathum S et al. Health-related quality of life as a predictor of mortality and hospitalization: The Dialysis Outcomes and Practice Patterns Study (DOPPS). *Kidney Int.* 2003 64:339-349

17. http://www.fda.gov/Drugs/DrugSafety/PostmarketDrugSafetyInformationforPatientsandProviders/ucm109375.htm. Accessed on July 21, 2011.

18. Singh AK, Szczech L, Tang KL, et al. Correction of anemia with epoetin alfa in chronic kidney disease. *N Engl J Med.* 2006 355(20):2085-2098

19. Schatell D, Witten B. Anemia: Dialysis patients' experiences. *Nephrol News Issues.* 2004. 18(12):49-54

20. Kutner N, Bowles T, Zhang R, et al. Dialysis facility characteristics and variation in employment rates: a national study. *Clin J Am Soc Nephrol.* 2008 3(1):111-6

21. U S Renal Data System, 2011 USRDS Annual Data Report: Atlas of Chronic Kidney Disease and End-Stage Renal Disease in the United States, National Institutes of Health, National Institute of Diabetes and Digestive and Kidney Diseases, Bethesda, MD, 2011.

22. Insurance Information Institute. How can I insure against loss of income? Accessed on July 21, 2011 at
http://www.iii.org/individuals/disability/lossofincome/

23. Blake C, Codd MB, Cassidy A, et al. Physical function, employment and quality of life in end-stage renal disease. *J Nephrol.* 2000 13(2):142-9

24. Kutner NG, Zhang R, Huang Y, et al. Depressed mood, usual activity level, and continued employment after starting dialysis. *Clin J Am Soc Nephrol.* 2010 5(11):2040-5

25. USRDS special data request, May 20, 2003. The data reported here were supplied by the United States Renal Data System (USRDS). The interpretation and reporting of these data are the responsibility of the author(s) and in no way should be seen as an official policy or interpretation of the U.S. government.

26. Guilloton S. Miami's KidneySpa treats dialysis patients with dignity, compassion and comfort. Accessed on July 21, 2011 at http://www.examiner.com/x-11804-Health-Care-Examiner~y2009m7d8-Miamis-KidneySpa-treats-dialysis-patients-with-dignity-compassion-and-comfort

27. Moore GE, Parsons DB, Stray-Gunderson J, et al. Uremic myopathy limits aerobic capacity in hemodialysis patients. *Am J Kidney Dis.* 1993 22(2):277-87

28. Sezer S, Elsurer R, Ulubay G, et al. Factors associated with peak oxygen uptake in hemodialysis patients awaiting renal transplantation. *Transplant Proc.* 2007 39(4):879-82

29. Brenner I, Brohart K. Weekly energy expenditure and quality of life in hemodialysis patients. *CANNT J.* 2008 18(4):36-40

30. Noori N, Kopple JD, Kovedsy CP, et al. Mid-arm muscle circumference and quality of life and survival in maintenance hemodialysis patients. *Clin J Am Soc Nephrol.* 2010 5(12):2258-68

31. Sun Y, Chen B, Jia Q, et al. [The effect of exercise during hemodialysis on adequacy of dialysis]. [Article in Chinese]. *Zhonghua Nei Ke Za Zhi.* 2002 41(2):79-81

32. Touissant ND, Polkinghorne KR, Kerr PG. Impact of intradialytic exercise on arterial compliance and B-type natriuretic peptide levels in hemodialysis patients. *Hemodial Int.* 2008 12(2):254-63

33. Farese S, Budmiger R, Aregger F, et al. Effect of trancutaneous electrical muscle stimulation and passive cycling movements on blood pressure and removal of urea and phosphate during hemodialysis. *Am J Kidney Dis.* 2008 52(4):745-52

34. Cheema B, Abas H, Smith B, et al. Progressive exercise for anabolism in kidney disease (PEAK): A randomized, controlled trial of resistance training during hemodialysis. *J Am Soc Nephrol.* 2007 18(5):1594-601

35. Yurtkuran M, Alp A, Yurtkuran M, et al. A modified yoga-based exercise program in hemodialysis patients: a randomized controlled study. *Complement Ther Med.* 15(3):164-71

36. Fiatarone MA, Marks EC, Ryan ND, et al. High-intensity strength training in nonagenarians. Effects on skeletal muscle. *JAMA.* 1990 263(22):3029-34

37. Basic-Jukic N, Juric I, Racki S, et al. Spontaneous tendon ruptures in patients with end-stage renal disease. *Kidney Blood Press Res.* 2009 32(1):32-6

38. Lai CF, Kao TW, Tsai TF, et al. Quantitative comparison of skin colors in patients with ESRD undergoing different dialysis modalities. *Am J Kidney Dis.* 2006 48(2):292-300

39. Masmoudi A, Ben Hmida M, Mseddi M, et al. [Cutaneous manifestations of chronic hemodialysis. Prospective study of 363 cases] [Article in French]. *Presse Med.* 35(3 Pt 1):399-406

40. Kshirsagar AV, Craig RG, Beck JD, et al. Severe periodontitis is associated with low serum albumin among patients on maintenance hemodialysis therapy. *Clin J Am Soc Nephrol.* 2007 2(2):239-44

41. Bots CP, Brand HS, Poorterman JH, et al. Oral and salivary changes in patients with end-stage renal disease (ESRD): a two-year follow-up study. *Br Dent J.* 2007 202(2):E3

42. Borawski J, Wilczynska-Borawska M, Stokowska W, et al. The periodontal status of pre-dialysis chronic kidney disease and maintenance dialysis patients. *Nephrol Dial Transplant.* 2007 22(2):457-64

43. Bayraktar G, Kurtulus I, Kazancioglu R, et al. Evaluation of periodontal parameters in patients undergoing peritoneal dialysis or hemodialysis. *Oral Dis.* 2008 14(2):185-9

44. AHA Guideline: Prevention of Infective Endocarditis. Accessed on July 21, 2011 at http://circ.ahajournals.org/cgi/reprint/CIRCULATIONAHA.106.183095

45. Mayo Clinic Staff. Dry mouth: Lifestyle and home remedies. Accessed on July 21, 2011 at http://www.mayoclinic.com/health/dry-mouth/HA00034/DSECTION=lifestyle%2Dand%2Dhome%2Dremedies

46. Accessed on July 21, 2011 at http://www.Quenchgum.com/html/nutritional_info.html#chunkinfo

47. Accessed on July 21, 2011 at http://www.biotene.com/

48. Frÿckstedt J, Hylander B. Sexual function in patients with end-stage renal disease. *Scand J Urol Nephrol.* 2008 42(5):466-71

49. Kettas E, Cayan F, Akbay E, et al. Sexual dysfunction and associated risk factors in women with end-stage renal disease. *J Sex Med.* 2008 5(4):872-7

50. Noohi S, Azar M, Behzadi AH, et al. Comparison of sexual function in females receiving hemodialysis and after transplantation. *J Ren Care.* 2010 36(4):212-7

51. Salvatierra O Jr, Fortmann JL, Belzer FO. Sexual function of males before and after renal transplantation. *Urology.* 1975. 5(1):64-6

52. Mahajan SK, Abbasi AA, Prasad AS, et al. Effects of oral zinc therapy on gonadal function in hemodialysis patients. A double-blind study. *Ann Intern Med.* 1982 97(3):357-61

53. Lawrence IG, Price DE, Howlett TA, et al. Correcting impotence in the male dialysis paitent: experience with testosterone replacement and vacuum tumescence therapy. *Am J Kidney Dis.* 1998 31(2):313-9

54. Beg S, Al-Khoury L, Cunningham GR. Testosterone replacement in men. *Curr Opion Endocrinol Diabetes Obes.* 2008 15(4):364-70

55. Snyder PJ, Peachey H, Berlin JA, et al. Effects of testosterone replacement in hypogonadal men. *J Clin Endocrinol Metab.* 2000 85(8):2670-7

56. Johansen KL. Testosterone metabolism and replacement therapy in patients with end-stage renal disease. *Semin Dial.* 2004 17(3):202-8

57. Brockenbrough AT, Dittrich MO, Page ST, et al. Transdermal androgen therapy to augment EPO in the treatment of anemia of chronic renal disease. *Am J Kidney Dis.* 2006 47(2):251-62

58. Punzo G, Maggi S, Ponzio R, et al. [Use of sildenafil in the chronic uremic patient] [Article in Italian]. *Minerva Urol Nephrol.* 2001 53(1):39-43

59. Chatterjee R, Wood S, McGarrigle HH, et al. A novel therapy with testosterone and sildenafil for erectile dysfunction in patients on renal dialysis or after renal transplantation. *J Fam Plan Reprod Health Care.* 2004 30(2):88-80

60. Bellinghieri G, Santoro G, Santoro D, et al. Ultrastructural changes of corpora cavernosa in men with erectile dysfunction and chronic renal failure. *Semin Nephrol.* 2004 (5):488-91

61. Schmidt RJ, Holley JL. Fertility and contraception in end-stage renal disease. *Adv Ren Replace Ther.* 1998 5(1):38-44

62. Reddy SS, Holley JL. The importance of increased dialysis and anemia management for infant survival in pregnant women on hemodialysis. *Kidney Int.* 2009 75(11):1133-4. Comment in *Kidney Int.* 2009 75(11):1217-22

63. Coyle M, Sulger E, Fletcher C, et al. A successful 39-week pregnancy on hemodialysis: A case report. *Nephrol Nurs J.* 2008 35(4):348-55, 402; quiz 356. Erratum in *Nephrol Nurs J.* 2008 35(5):489

64. Barua M, Hladunewich M, Keunen J, et al. Successful pregnancies on nocturnal home hemodialysis. *Clin J Am Soc Nephrol.* 2008 3(2):392-6. Comment in *Clin J Am Soc Nephrol.* 2008 3(2):312-3

65. Ferrannini M, Vischini G, Miani N, et al. Successful pregnancy in a uremic patient treated with single needle hemodialysis. *Int J Artif Organs.* 2007 30(12):1122-5

66. Abd KH, Al-Shamma I. Successful pregnancy in a patient with hemodialysis in Iraq. *Saudi J Kidney Dis Transpl.* 2007 18(2):257-60

67. Bamberg C, Diekmann F, Haase M, et al. Pregnancy on intensified hemodialysis: fetal surveillance and perinatal outcome. *Fetal Diagn Ther.* 2007 22(4):289-93

68. Allada R, Siegel JM. Unearthing the phylogenetic roots of sleep. *Curr Biol.* 2008 18(15):R670-R679

69. Smith M, Segal R. How much sleep do you need? Accessed on July 21, 2011 at http://www.helpguide.org/life/sleeping.htm

70. Kerkhofs M, Boudjeltia KZ, Stenuit P, et al. Sleep restriction increases blood neutrophils, total chelesterol and low density lipprotein cholesterol in postmenopausal women: A preliminary study. *Maturitas.* 2007 56(2):212-5

71. Chaput JP, Despres JP, Bouchard C, et al. The association between sleep duration and weight gain in adults: a 6-year prospective study from the Quebec Family Study. *Sleep.* 2008 31(4):517-23

72. Tuomilehto H, Peltonen M, Partinen M, et al. Sleep duration is associated with an increased risk for the prevalence of type 2 diabetes in middle-aged wome – the FIN-D2D survey. *Sleep Med.* 2008 9(3):221-7. Comment in *Sleep Med.* 2008 9(3):219-20

73. Philip P, Sagaspe P, Taillard J, et al. Fatigue, sleepiness, and performance in simulated versus real driving conditions. *Sleep.* 2005 28(12):1511-6

74. Jansson-Frojmark M, Lindblom K. A bidirectional relationship between anxiety and depression, and insomnia? A prospective study in the general population. *J Psychosom Res.* 2008 64(4):443-9

75. Hornung OP, Regen F, Danker-Hopfe H, et al. The relationship between REM sleep and memory consolidation in old age and effects of cholinergic medication. *Biol Psychiatry.* 2007 61(6):750-7

76. Elder SJ, Pisoni RL, Akizawa T, et al. Sleep quality predicts quality of life and mortality risk in haemodialysis patients: results from the Dialysis Outcomes and Practice Patterns Study (DOPPS). *Nephrol Dial Transplant.* 2008 23(3):998-1004

77. Davison SN, Jhangri GS. The impact of chronic pain on depression, sleep, and the desire to withdraw from dialysis in hemodialysis patients. *J Pain Symptom Manage.* 2005 30(5):465-73

78. Pisoni RL, Wikstrom B, Elder SJ, et al. Pruritus in haemodialysis patients: International results from the Dialysis Outcomes and Practice Patterns Study (DOPPS). *Nephrol Dial Transplant.* 2006 21(12):3495-505. Comment in *Nephrol Dial Transplant.* 2007 22(12):3669-70

79. Hsu CY, Lee CT, Lee YJ, et al. Better sleep quality and less daytime symptoms in patients on evening hemodialysis: a questionnaire-based study. *Artif Organs.* 2008 32(9):711-6

80. Bastos JP, Sousa RB, Nepomuceno LA, et al. Sleep disturbances in patients on maintenance hemodialysis: role of dialysis shift. *Rev Assoc Med Bras.* 2007 53(6):492-6

81. Parker KP, Bailey JL, Rye DB, et al. Insomnia on dialysis nights: the beneficial effects of cool dialysate. *J Nephrol.* 2008 21 Suppl 13:S71-7

82. U S Renal Data System, USRDS 2009 Annual Data Report: Atlas of Chronic Kidney Disease and End-Stage Renal Disease in the United States, Table H.12. National Institutes of Health, National Institute of Diabetes and Digestive and Kidney Diseases, Bethesda, MD, 2009.

83. Wingard R. Reducing early mortality in patients on dialysis: lessons from the RightStart program. *Nephrol Nurs J.* 2009 36(2):215-20

84. http://www.reuters.com/article/pressRelease/idUS16647+30-Mar-2009+PRN20090330 Accessed July 21, 2011

85. Gotch FA, Levin NW. Daily dialysis: the long and the short of it. *Blood Purif.* 2003 21(4-5):271-81

86. Twardowski ZJ. Short, thrice-weekly hemodialysis is inadequate regardless of small molecule clearance. *ASAIO J.* 2004 27(6):452-66

Chapter 7

1. Tsay SL, Hung LO. Empowerment of patients with end-stage renal disease--a randomized controlled trial. *Int J Nurs Stud.* 2004 41(1):59-65

2. Tovbin D, Gidron Y, Jean T, et al. Relative importance and interrelations between psychosocial factors and individualized quality of life of hemodialysis patients. *Qual Life Res.* 2003 12(6):709-17

3. Tsay SL, Healstead M. Self-care self-efficacy, depression, and quality of life among patients receiving dialysis in Taiwan. *Int J Nurs Stud.* 2002 39(3):245-51

4. U S Renal Data System, 2011 USRDS Annual Data Report: Atlas of Chronic Kidney Disease and End-Stage Renal Disease in the United States, National Institutes of Health, National Institute of Diabetes and Digestive and Kidney Diseases, Bethesda, MD, 2011.

5. Povlsen JV, Ivarsen P. How to start the late referred ESRD patient urgently on chronic APD. *Nephrol Dial Transplant.* 2006 21 Suppl 2:ii56-9

6. The "bathtub" (presternal) PD catheter. Accessed on July 21, 2011 at http://www.homedialysis.org/article/life_at_home/the_bathtub_presternal_pd_catheter

7. Rabindranath KS, Adams J, Ali TZ, et al. Automated vs. continuous ambulatory peritoneal dialysis: a systematic review of randomized controlled trials. *Nephrol Dial Transplant.* 2007 22(10):2991-8

8. Bargman JM. Tailoring automated PD (APD) to your life. Home Dialysis Central, May, 2008 http://www.homedialysis.org/resources/tom/200805/

9. What is a peritoneal equilibration test? Accessed on July 21, 2011 at http://www.kidney.org.uk/Medical-Info/pd/pet_test.html

10. Stack AG. Determinants of modality selection among incident US dialysis patients: Results from a national study. *J Am Soc Nephrol.* 2002 13:1279-1287

11. Schreiber M, Ilamathi E, Wolfson M, et al. Preliminary findings from the National pre-ESRD Education Initiative. *Nephrol News Issues.* 2000 14(12):44-6

12. Mehrotra R, Marsh D, Vonesh E, et al. Patient education and access of ESRD patients to renal replacement therapies beyond in-center hemodialysis. *Kidney Int.* 2005 68:378-390

13. Berger M. Performing CAPD independently with one hand using an assist device. *ANNA J.* 1996 23(6):618-22

14. Baxter EZ-AIDE assist device. Accessed July 21, 2011 at http://www.ecomm.baxter.com/ecatalog/browseCatalog.do?lid=10001&hid=10001&cid=10016&key=fb2e98eed78cc513e27a3aaa6c2ed63&pid=458291 Accessed May 22, 2007.

15. Schuetz CE. Training a continuous ambulatory peritoneal dialysis patient with one functional arm. *Adv Perit Dial.* 2005 21:146-7

16. Lambert MC, Lage C, Kirchgessner J. Stay.safe. A new PVC free system in long-term CAPD treatment. *EDTNA ERCA J.* 1999 25(3):30-4

17. Flynn CT. Why blind diabetics with renal failure should be offered treatment. *Br Med J (Clin Res Ed).* 1983 287(6400):1177-8

18. Wright LS. Training a patient with visual impairment on continuous ambulatory peritoneal dialysis. *Nephrol Nurs J.* 2005 32(6):675,666

19. Bentley ML. Keep it simple! A touch technique peritoneal dialysis procedure for the blind and visually impaired. *CANNT J.* 2001 11(2):32-4. Comment in: *CANNT J.* 2001 11(4):8

20. Pietrzak B, Olszowska A, Wankowicz Z. [Continuous ambulatory peritoneal dialysis as a renal replacement therapy in blind diabetics with type 1 diabetes] [Article in Polish] *Pol Merkur Lekarski.* 1998 (29):271-3

21. Chandran PK, Lane T, Flynn CT. Patient and technique survival for blind and sighted diabetics on continuous ambulatory peritoneal dialysis: a ten-year analysis. *Int J Artif Organs.* 1991 14(5):262-8

22. Kushner A. Adaptation of the Fresenius PD+ Cycler for a hearing-impaired patient. *Adv Perit Dial.* 2000 16:163-4

23. Winchester JF. Peritoneal dialysis in older individuals. *Geriatr Nephrol Urol.* 1999 9(3):147-52

24. Teitelbaum I. Peritoneal dialysis is appropriate for elderly patients. *Contrib Nephrol.* 2006 150:240-6

25. Dimkovic N, Oreopoulos DG. Chronic peritoneal dialysis in the elderly: a review. *Perit Dial Int.* 2000 20(3):276-83

26. Dimkovic NB, Prakash S, Roscoe J, et al. Chronic peritoneal dialysis in octogenarians. *Nephrol Dial Transplant.* 2001 16(10):2034-40

27. Sunder S, Taskapan H, Jojoa J, et al. Chronic peritoneal dialysis in the tenth decade of life. *Int Urol Nephrol.* 2004 36(4):605-9

28. Twardowski ZJ. Presternal peritoneal catheter. *Adv Ren Replace Ther.* 2002 9(2):125-32

29. McDonald SP, Collins JF, Rumpsfeld M, et al. Obesity is a risk factor for peritonitis in the Australian and New Zealand peritoneal dialysis patient populations. *Perit Dial Int.* 2004 24(4):340-6

30. Aslam N, Bernardini J, Fried L, et al. Large body mass index does not predict short-term survival in peritoneal dialysis patients. *Perit Dial Int.* 2002 22(2):191-6 Comment in: *Perit Dial Int.* 2002 22(5):634-5; author reply 635-6.

31. McDonald SP, Collins JF, Johnson DW. Obesity is associated with worse peritoneal dialysis outcomes in the Australia and New Zealand patient populations. *J Am Soc Nephrol.* 2003 14(11):2894-901

32. Vonesh EF, Snyder JJ, Foley RN, et al. Mortality studies comparing peritoneal dialysis and hemodialysis: what do they tell us? *Kidney Int Suppl.* 2006 Nov;(103):S3-11

33. Garcia-Urena MA, Rodriguez CR, Vega Ruiz V, et al. Prevalence and management of hernias in peritoneal dialysis patients. *Perit Dial Int.* 2006 26(2):198-202. Comment in: *Perit Dial Int.* 2006 26(2):178-82

34. Johns EM, Poole G. Gs20p single-centre experience with mesh repair of abdominal hernia in CAPD patients. *ANZ J Surg.* 2007 77 Suppl 1:A30

35. Shah H, Chu M, Bargman JM. Perioperative management of peritoneal dialysis patients undergoing hernia surgery without the use of interim hemodialysis. *Perit Dial Int.* 2006 26(6):684-7

36. Manley HJ, Garvin CG, Drayer DK, et al. Medication prescribing patterns in ambulatory haemodialysis patients: comparisons of USRDS to a large not-for-profit dialysis provider. *Nephrol Dial Transplant.* 2004 19:1842-1848

37. Szeto CC, Chow KM, Kwan BC, et al. Relation between number of prescribed medication and outcome in peritoneal dialysis patients. *Clin Nephrol.* 2006 66(4):256-62

38. Boudville NC, Cordy P, Millman K, et al. Blood pressure, volume and sodium control in an automated peritoneal dialysis population. *Perit Dial Int.* 2007 27(5):537-43

39. Dong J, Wang H, Wang M. Low prevalence of hyperphosphatemia independent of residual renal function in peritoneal dialysis patients. *J Ren Nutr.* 2007 17(6):389-96

40. Witten B, Schatell DR, Becker BN. Relationship of ESRD working-age patient employment to treatment modality. Poster presented at the American Society of Nephrology meeting, St. Louis, MO, October 31, 2004. (Abstract) *J Am Soc Nephrol.* 2004 15:633A.

41. Snyder JJ, Kasiske BL, Gilbertson DT, et al. A comparison of transplant outcomes in peritoneal and hemodialysis patients. *Kidney Int.* 62(4):1423-30, 2002

42. U.S. Department of Transportation. 14 cfr part 382: Nondiscrimination on the Basis of Disability in Air Travel. Accessed on July 21, 2011 at http://www.southwest.com/assets/pdfs/customer_service/14cfr_part382.pdf

43. What Airline Employees, Airline Contractors, and Air Travelers with Disabilities Need to Know About Access to Air Travel for Persons with Disabilities: A Guide to the Air Carrier Access Act (ACAA) and its implementing regulations 14 CFR part 382 (page 8). Accessed on July 21, 2011 at http://airconsumer.ost.dot.gov/legislation/acaa/TAM-07-15-05.pdf

44. U.S. Department of Transportation. Section 382.57 of 14 CFR Part 382 reads "Charges for accommodations prohibited. Carriers shall not impose charges for providing facilities, equipment, or services that are required by this part to be provided to qualified individuals with a disability." Accessed on July 21, 2011 at http://www.gpo.gov/fdsys/pkg/CFR-2009-title14-vol4/xml/CFR-2009-title14-vol4-part382.xml#seqnum382.57

45. What Airline Employees, Airline Contractors, and Air Travelers with Disabilities Need to Know About Access to Air Travel for Persons with Disabilities: A Guide to the Air Carrier Access Act (ACAA) and its implementing regulations, 14 CFR Part 382 (Part 382). Accessed July 21, 2011 at http://airconsumer.dot.gov/legislation/acaa/TAM-07-15-05.pdf. Appendix III: Frequently Asked Questions. Page 147

46. Stack AG, Murthy B. Exercise and limitations in physical activity levels among new dialysis patients in the United States: an epidemiologic study. *Ann Epidemiol.* 2008 18(12):880-8

47. Lee SJ, Yoo JS. [The effects of a physical activity reinforcement program on exercise compliance, depression, and anxiety in continuous ambulatory peritoneal dailysis patients. [Article in Korean] *Taehan Kanho Hakhoe Chi.* 2004 34(3):440-8

48. Kettas E, Cayan F, Akbay E, et al. Sexual dysfunction and associated risk factors in women with end-stage renal disease. *J Sex Med.* 2008 5(4):872-7

49. Basok EK, Atsu N, Rifaioglu MM, et al. Assessment of female sexual function and quality of life in predialysis, peritoneal dialysis, hemodialysis, and renal transplant patients. *Int Urol Nephrol.* 2009 41(3):473-81

50. Lai CF, Wang Yt, Hung KY, et al. Sexual dysfunction in peritoneal dialysis patients. *Am J Nephrol.* 2007 27(6):615-21

51. Dachille G, Pagliarulo V, Ludovico GM, et al. Sexual dysfunction in patients under dialytic treatment. *Minerva Urol Nefrol.* 2006 58(2):195-200

52. YenicerioGlu Y, Kefi A, Aslan G, et al. Efficacy and safety of sildenafil for treating erectile dysfunction in patients on dialysis. *BJU Int.* 2002 90(4):442-5

53. Hosfield EM, Rabban JT, Chen LM, et al. Squamous metaplasia of the ovarian surface epithelium and subsurface fibrosis: distinctive pathologic fndings in the ovaries and fallopian tubes of patients on peritoneal dialysis. *Int J Gynecol Pathol.* 2008 27(4):465-74

54. Jefferys A, Wyburn K, Chow J, et al. Peritoneal dialysis in pregnancy: a case series. *Nephrology (Carlton).* 2008 13(5):380-3

55. Vazquez AFG, Calva IEM, Fernandez RM, et al. Pregnancy in end-stage renal disease patients and treatment with peritoneal dialysis: report of two cases. *Perit Dial Int.* 2007 27:353-8

56. Chou CY, Ting IW, Lin TH, et al. Pregnancy in patients on chronic dialysis: a single center experience and combined analysis of reported results. *Eur J Obstet Gynecol Reprod Biol.* 2008 136(2):165-70

57. Eryavuz N, Yuksel S, Acarturk G, et al. Comparison of sleep quality between hemodialysis and peritoneal dialysis patients. *Int Urol Nephrol.* 2008 40(3):785-91

58. Guney I, Biyik M, Yeksan M, et al. Sleep quality and depression in peritoneal dialysis patients. *Ren Fail.* 2008 30(10):1017-22

59. Tang SC, Lam B, Ku PP, et al. Alleviation of sleep apnea in patients with chronic renal failure by nocturnal cycler-assisted peritoneal dialysis compared with conventional continuous ambulatory peritoneal dialysis. *J Am Soc Nephrol.* 2006 17(9):2607-16

60. Chandna SM, Farrington K. Residual renal function: Considerations on its importance and preservation in dialysis patients. *Sem Dial.* 2004 17(3):196-201

61. Maiorca R, Brunori G, Zubani R, et al. Predictive value of dialysis adequacy and nutritional indices for mortality and morbidity in CAPD and HD patients. A longitudinal study. *Nephrol Dial Transplant.* 1995 10(12):2295-305

62. Termorshuizen F, Korevaar JC, Dekker FW, et al. The relative importance of residual renal function compared with peritoneal clearance for patient survival and quality of life: An analysis of the Netherlands Cooperative Study on the Adequacy of Dialysis (NECOSAD)-2. *Am J Kidney Dis.* 2003 41(6):1293-1302

63. Horinek A, Misra M. Does residual renal function decline more rapidly in hemodialysis than in peritoneal dialysis? How good is the evidence? *Adv Perit Dial.* 2004 20:137-40

64. Misra M, Vonesh E, Churchill N, et al. Preservation of glomerular filtration rate on dialysis when adjusted for patient dropout. *Kidney Int.* 2000 57(2):691-6

65. Misra M, Vonesh E, Van Stone JC, et al. Effect of cause and time of dropout on the residual GFR: A comparative analysis of the decline of GFR on dialysis. *Kidney Int.* 2001 59(2):754-63

66. Shin SK, Noh H, Kang SW, et al. Risk factors influencing the decline of residual renal function in continuous ambulatory peritoneal dialysis patients. *Perit Dial Int.* 1999 19(2):138-42

67. Rocco M, Burkart JM. Abdominal hernias in continuous peritoneal dialysis. Accessed July 21, 2011 at http://www.uptodate.com/patients/content/topic.do?topicKey=dialysis/18539

68. Harel Z, Wald R, Bell C, et al. Outcome of patients who develop early-onset peritonitis. *Adv Perit Dial.* 2006 22:46-9

69. Balasubramaniam G, Brown EA, Davenport A, et al. The Pan-Thames EPS study: treatment and outcomes of encapsulating peritoneal sclerosis. *Nephrol Dial Transplant.* 2009 24(10):3209-15

70. Kropp J, Sinsakul M, Butsch J, et al. Laparoscopy in the early diagnosis and management of sclerosing encapsulating peritonitis. *Semin Dial.* 2009 22(3):304-7

71. Johnson DW, Cho Y, Livingston BE, et al. Encapsulating peritoneal sclerosis: incidence, predictors, and outcomes. *Kidney Int.* 2010 77(10):904-12

72. Lo WK, Kawanishi H. Encapsulating peritoneal sclerosis—medical and surgical treatment. *Perit Dial Int.* 2009 29 Suppl 2:S211-4

73. Ireton-Jones C. *Handbook of Home Nutrition Support.* Jones and Bartlett, 2007. Boston, Toronto, London, Singapore

74. Inrig JK, Sun JL, Yang Q, et al. Mortality by dialysis modality among patients who have end-stage renal disease and are awaiting renal transplantation. *Clin J Am Soc Nephrol.* 2006 1(4):774-9

75. Mehrotra R. Long-term outcomes in automated peritoneal dialysis: similar or better than in continuous ambulatory peritoneal dialysis? *Perit Dial Int.* 2009 29 Suppl 2:S111-4

76. Jaar BG, Coresh J, Plantinga LC, et al. Comparing the risk for death with peritoneal dialysis and hemodialysis in a national cohort of patients with chronic kidney disease. *Ann Intern Med.* 2005 143(3):174-83. Comment in *Ann Intern Med.* 2005 143(3):229-31

77. Twardowski ZJ, Moore HL, Prowant BF, et al. Long-term follow-up of body size indices, residual kidney function, and peritoneal transport characteristics in continuous ambulatory peritoneal dialysis. *Adv Perit Dial.* 2009 25:155-64

Chapter 8

1. Home Dialysis Central tracking. December, 2011. Medical Education Institute, Inc.

2. Lockridge RS, Moran J. Short daily hemodialysis and nocturnal hemodialysis at home: practical considerations. *Semin Dial.* 2008 20(1):49-53

3. Goldfarb-Rumyantzev AS, Cheung AK, Leypoldt JK. Computer simulation of small-solute and middle-molecule removal during short daily and long thrice-weekly hemodialysis. *Am J Kidney Dis.* 2002 40(6):1211-8

4. Piccoli GB, Bermond F, Mezza E, et al. Vascular access survival and morbidity on daily dialysis: a comparative analysis of home and limited care haemodialysis. *Nephrol Dial Transplant.* 2004 19(8):2084-94

5. The FHN Trial Group. In-center hemodialysis six times per week versus three times per week. *N Engl J Med.* 2010 363:2287-2300

6. Wise M, Schatell D, Klicko K, et al. Successful daily home hemodialysis patient-care partner dyads: benefits outweigh burdens. *Hemodial Int.* 2010 14(3):278-88

7. Kumar VA, Ledezma ML, Rasgon SA. Daily home hemodialysis at a health maintenance organization: three-year experience. *Hemodial Int.* 2007 11(2):225-30

8. He Q, Chen J, Xu Y, et al. High-risk end-stage renal disease patients converted from conventional to short daily haemodialysis. *J Int Med Res.* 2006 34(6):682-8

9. Yuen D, Richardson RM, Chan CT. Improvements in phosphate control with short daily in-center hemodialysis. *Clin Nephrol.* 2005 64(5):364-70

10. Fagugli RM, Reboldi G, Quintaliani G, et al. Short daily hemodialysis: blood pressure control and left ventricular mass reduction in hypertensive hemodialysis patients. *Am J Kidney Dis.* 2001 38(2):371-6

11. Ting GO, Kjellstrang C, Freitas T, et al. Long-term study of high-comorbidity ESRD patients converted from conventional to short daily hemodialysis. *Am J Kidney Dis.* 2003 42(5):1020-35

12. Painter P, Krasnoff JB, Kuskowski M, et al. Effects of modality change and transplant on peak oxygen uptake in patients with kidney failure. *Am J Kidney Dis.* 2011 57(1):113-22

13. Ettari G, Boccardo G, De Prisco O, et al. [Daily short dialysis. First results in a group of patients in home dialysis training.] *Minerva Urol Nefrol.* 2002 54(2):139-43 [Article in Italian]

14. Coyle M, Sulger E, Fletcher C, et al. A successful 39-week pregnancy on hemodialysis: A case report. *Nephrol Nurs J.* 2008 35(4):348-55, 402; quiz 356. Erratum in *Nephrol Nurs J.* 2008 35(5):489

15. Ferrannini M, Vischini G, Miani N, et al. Successful pregnancy in a uremic patient treated with single needle hemodialysis. *Int J Artif Organs.* 2007 30(12):1122-5

16. Abd KH, Al-Shamma I. Successful pregnancy in a patient with hemodialysis in Iraq. *Saudi J Kidney Dis Transpl.* 2007 18(2):257-60

17. Bamberg C, Diekmann F, Haase M, et al. Pregnancy on intensified hemodialysis: fetal surveillance and perinatal outcome. *Fetal Diagn Ther.* 2007 22(4):289-93

18. Jaber BL, Schiller B, Burkart JM, et al; FREEDOM Study Group. Impact of short daily hemodialysis on restless legs symptoms and sleep disturbances. *Clin J Am Soc Nephrol.* 2011 6(5):1049-56. Epub 2011 Mar 17.

19. Lugon JR, Andre MB. Initial Brazilian experience with short-duration in-center daily hemodialysis. *Hemodial Int.* 2005 9(1):3-6

20. Goldfarb-Rumyantzev AS, Leypoldt JK, Nelson N, et al. A crossover study of short daily hemodialysis. *Nephrol Dial Transplant.* 2006 21(1):166-75

21. Williams AW, Chebrolu SB, Ing TS, et al; Daily Hemodialysis Study Group. *Am J Kidney Dis.* 2004 43(1):90-102

22. Jaber BL, Lee Y, Collins AJ, et al.; FREEDOM Study Group. Effect of daily hemodialysis on depressive symptoms and post-dialysis recovery time: interim report from the FREEDOM (Following Rehabilitation, Economics, and Everyday Dialysis Outcomes Measurements) Study. *Am J Kidney Dis.* 2010 56(3):531-9

23. Nesrallah G, Suri R, Moist L, et al. Volume control and blood pressure management in patients undergoing quotidian dialysis. *Am J Kidney Dis.* 2003 42(1 Suppl):13-7

24. Okada K, Abe M, Hagi C, et al. Prolonged protective effect of short daily hemodialysis against dialysis-induced hypotension. *Kidney Blood Press Res.* 2005 28(2):68-76

25. Ayus JC, Mizani MR, Achinger SG, et al. Effects of short daily versus conventional hemodialysis on left ventricular hypertrophy and inflammatory markers: a prospective controlled study. *J Am Soc Nephrol.* 2005 16(9):2778-88

26. Traeger J, Galland R, Delawari E, et al. Six years' experience with short daily hemodialysis: do the early improvements persist in the mid and long term? *Hemodial Int.* 2004 8(2):151-8

27. Suri R, Depner TA, Blake PG, et al. Adequacy of quotidian hemodialysis. *Am J Kidney Dis.* 2003 42(1 Suppl):42-8

28. Goldfarb-Rumyantzev AS, Cheung AK, Leypoldt JK. Computer simulation of small-solute and middle-molecule removal during short daily and long thrice-weekly hemodialysis. *Am J Kidney Dis.* 2002 40(6):1211-8

29. Fagugli RM, De Smet R, Buoncristiani U, et al. Behavior of non-protein-bound and protein-bound uremic solutes during daily hemodialysis. *Am J Kidney Dis.* 2002 40(2):339-47

30. Galland R, Traeger J, Arkouche W, et al. Short daily hemodialysis rapidly improves nutritional status in hemodialysis patients. *Kidney Int.* 2001 60(4):1555-60

31. Galland R, Traeger J, Arkouche W, et al. Short daily hemodialysis and nutritional status. *Am J Kidney Dis.* 2001 37(1 Suppl 2):S95-8

32. Galland R, Traeger J. Short daily hemodialysis and nutritional status in patients with chronic renal failure. *Semin Dial.* 2004 17(2):104-8

33. Lowrie EG, Curtin RB, LePain N, et al. Medical Outcomes Study Short Form-36: A consistent and powerful predictor of morbidity and mortality in dialysis patients. *Am J Kidney Dis.* 2003 41:1286-1291

34. Heidenheim AP, Muirhead N, Moist L, et al. Patient quality of life on quotidian hemodialysis. *Am J Kidney Dis.* 2003 42(1 Suppl):36-41

35. Leypoldt JK, Cheung AK, Deeter RB, et al. Kinetics of urea and beta-microglobulin during and after short hemodialysis treatments. *Kidney Int.* 2004 66(4):1669-76

36. Martins Castro MC, Luders C, Elias RM, et al. High-efficiency short daily haemodialysis—morbidity and mortality rate in a long-term study. *Nephrol Dial Transplant.* 2006 21(8):2232-8

37. Kjellstrand CM, Buoncristiani U, Ting G, et al. Short daily hemodialysis: survival in 415 patients treated for 1006 patient years. *Nephrol Dial Transplant.* 2008 23(10);3283-8

Chapter 9

1. Agar JW, Somerville CA, Dwyer KM, et al. Nocturnal hemodialysis in Australia. *Hemodial Int.* 2003 7(4):278-89

2. Agar JW, Knight RJ, Simmonds RE, et al. Nocturnal haemodialysis: an Australian cost comparison with conventional satellite haemodialysis. *Nephrology (Carlton).* 2005 10(6):557-70

3. Lockridge RS, Moran J. Short daily hemodialysis and nocturnal hemodialysis at home: practical considerations. *Semin Dial.* 2008 20(1):49-53

4. Accessed July 21, 2011 at http://www.hemausa.com/. Accessed July 21, 2011 at http://www.tntmoborg.com/immobile.html

5. Lindsay RM, Heidenheim PA, Nesrallah G, et al. Daily Hemodialysis Study Group London Health Sciences Center. Minutes to recovery after a hemodialysis session: a simple health-related quality of life question that is reliable, valid, and sensitive to change. *Clin J Am Soc Nephrol.* 2006 1(5):952-9

6. Jefferies HJ, Virk B, Schiller B, et al. Frequent hemodialysis schedules are associated with reduced levels of dialysis-induced cardiac injury (myocardial stunning). *Clin J Am Soc Nephrol.* 2011 6(6):1326-32

7. Nagase S, Hirayama A, Ueda A, et al. Light-shielded hemodialysis prevents hypotension and lipid peroxidation by inhibiting nitric oxide production. *Clin Chem.* 2005 51:2397-8

8. Kooienga L. Phosphorus balance with daily dialysis. *Semin Dial.* 2007 20(4):342-5

9. Toissant N, Boddington J, Simmonds R, et al. Calcium phosphate metabolism and bone mineral density with nocturnal hemodialysis. *Hemodial Int.* 2006 10(3):280-6

10. Sikkes ME, Kooistra MP, Weijs PJM. Improved nutrition after conversion to nocturnal home hemodialysis. *J Renal Nutr.* 2009 19(6):494-9

11. Micha R, Mozaffarian D. Trans fatty acids: effects on metabolic syndrome, heart disease and diabetes. *Nat Rev Endocrinol.* 2009 Jun;5(6):335-44

12. Pierratos A, Ouwendyk M, Francoeur R, et al. Nocturnal hemodialysis: three-year experience. *J Am Soc Nephrol.* 1998 9(5):859-68. Comment in *J Am Soc Nephrol.* 1998 9(5):899-900

13. Schwartz DI, Pierratos A, Richardson RM, et al. Impact of nocturnal home hemodialysis on anemia management in patients with end-stage renal disease. *Clin Nephrol.* 2005 63(3):202-8

14. Klarenback S, Heidenheim AP, Leitch R, et al; Daily/Nocturnal Dialysis Study Group. Reduced requirement for erythropoietin with quotidian hemodialysis therapy. *ASAIO J.* 2002 48(1):57-61

15. Chan CT, Liu PP, Arab S, et al. Nocturnal hemodialysis improves erythropoietin responsiveness and growth of hematopoietic stem cells. *J Am Soc Nephrol.* 2009 20(3):665-71

16. Bergman A, Fenton SS, Richardson RM, et al. Reduction in cardiovascular related hospitalization with nocturnal home hemodialysis. *Clin Nephrol.* 2008 69(1):33-9

17. Chan CT, Notarius CF, Merlocco AC, et al. Improvement in exercise duration and capacity after conversion to nocturnal home haemodialysis. *Nephrol Dial Transplant.* 2007 22(11):3285-91

18. Personal communication with John Moran, MD. Slide of unpublished data provided via email on 6/10/09

19. Gangji AS, Windrim R, Gandhi S, et al. Successful pregnancy with nocturnal hemodialysis. *Am J Kidney Dis.* 2004 44(5):912-6

20. Barua M, Hladunewich M, Keunen J, et al. Successful pregnancies on nocturnal home hemodialysis. *Clin J Am Soc Nephrol.* 2008 3(2):392-6. Comment in *Clin J Am Soc Nephrol.* 2008 3(2):312-3

21. Koch BC, Nagtegaal JE, Hagen EC, et al. Different melatonin rhythrms and sleep-wake rhythms in patients on peritoneal dialysis, daytime hemodialysis, and nocturnal hemodialysis. *Sleep Med.* 2010 11(3):242-6

22. Beecroft JM, Duffin J, Pierratos A, et al. Decreased chemosensitivity and improvement of sleep apnea by nocturnal hemodialysis. *Sleep Med.* 2009 10(1):47-54. Comment in *Sleep Med.* 2009 10(1):15-8

23. Beecroft JM, Hoffstein V, Pierratos A, et al. Nocturnal haemodialysis increases pharyngeal size in patients with sleep apnoea and end-stage renal disease. *Nephrol Dial Transplant.* 2008 23(2):673-9

24. Hinghofer-Szalkay H. [Investigations concerning postural influence on blood and blood plasma (author's transl)] [Article in German]. *Klin Wochenschr.* 1980 58(20):1147-54

25. David S, Kumpers P, Eisenbach GM, et al. Prospective evaluation of an in-centre conversion from conventional haemodialysis to an intensified nocturnal strategy. *Nephrol Dial Transplant.* 2009 24(7):2232-40

26. Chan CT, Harvey PJ, Picton P, et al. Short-term blood pressure, noradrenergic, and vascular effects of nocturnal home hemodialysis. *Hypertension.* 2003 42(5):925-31

27. Chan C, Floras JS, Miller JA, et al. Improvement in ejection fraction by nocturnal haemodialysis in end-stage renal failure patients with coexisting heart failure. *Nephrol Dial Transplant.* 2002 17(8):1518-21

28. Chan CT, Shen XS, Picton P, et al. Nocturnal home hemodialysis improves baroreflex effectiveness index of end-stage renal disease patients. *J Hypertens.* 2008 26(9):1795-800

29. Chan CT, Floras JS, Miller JA, et al. Regression of left ventricular hypertrophy after conversion to nocturnal hemodialysis. *Kidney Int.* 2002 61(6):2235-9

30. Culleton BF, Walsh M, Klarenbach SW, et al. Effect of frequent nocturnal hemodialysis vs conventional hemodialysis on left ventricular mass and quality of life: a randomized controlled trial. *JAMA.* 2007 298(11):1291-9. Comment in *JAMA* 2007 298(11):1331-3, *Semin Dial.* 2008 21(2):192-5

31. Chan CT, Mardirossian S, Faratro R, et al. Improvement in lower-extremity peripheral arterial disease by nocturnal hemodialysis. *Am J Kidney Dis.* 41(1):225-9

32. Goldfarb-Rumyantzev AS, Cheung AK, Leypoldt JK. Computer simulation of small-solute and middle-molecule removal during short daily and long thrice-weekly hemodialysis. *Am J Kidney Dis.* 2002 40(6):1211-8

33. Nessim SJ, Jassal SV, Fung SV, et al. Conversion from conventional to nocturnal hemodialysis improves vitamin D levels. *Kidney Int.* 2007 71(11):1172-6

34. Yuen D, Richardson RM, Fenton SS, et al. Quotidian nocturnal hemodialysis improves cytokine profile and enhances erythropoietin responsiveness. *ASAIO J.* 2005 51(3):236-41

35. Bugeja AL, Chan CT. Improvement in lipid profile by nocturnal hemodialysis in patients with end-stage renal disease. *ASAIO J.* 2004 50(4):328-31

36. Van Eps CL, Jeffries JK, Anderson JA, et al. Mineral metabolism, bone histomorphometry and vascular calcification in alternate night nocturnal hemodialysis. *Nephrology (Carlton).* 2007 12(13):224-33

37. Kim SJ, Goldstein M, Szabo T, et al. Resolution of massive uremic tumoral calcinosis with daily nocturnal hemodialysis. *Nephrology (Carlton).* 2007 12(3):224-33

38. Jassal SV, Devins GM, Chan CT, et al. Improvements in cognition in patients converting from thrice weekly hemodialysis to nocturnal hemodialysis: a longitudinal pilot study. *Kidney Int.* 2006 70(5):956-62

39. Charra B, Calemard E, Ruffet M, et al. Survival as an index of quality of dialysis. *Kidney Int.* 1992 41:1286-1291

40. Pauly RP, Gill JS, Rose CL, et al. Survival among nocturnal home haemodialysis patients compared to kidney transplant recipients. *Nephrol Dial Transplant.* 2009 24(9):2915-9

41. Johansen KL, Zhang R, Huang Y, et al. Survival and hospitalization among patients using nocturnal and short daily compared to conventional hemodialysis: a USRDS study. *Kidney Int.* 2009 76(9):984-90

42. Lockridge RS, Kjellstrand CM. Nightly home hemodialysis: outcomes and factors associated with survival. *Hemodial Int.* 2011 15(2):211-8

43. Cafazzo JA, Leonard K, Easty AC, et al. Patient-perceived barriers to the adoption of nocturnal home hemodialysis. *Clin J Am Soc Nephrol.* 2009 4(4):784-9. Comment in *Clin J Am Soc Nephrol.* 2009 4(4):694-5

Chapter 10

No references

Chapter 11

No references

Chapter 12

1. Accessed on July 22, 2011 at http://www.medicare.gov/Dialysis/static/incDialysisCareCenters_Text.asp

2. Method to Assess Treatment Choices for Home Dialysis (MATCH-D). Home Dialysis Central. Accessed on July 22, 2011 at http://www.homedialysis.org/MATCH-D

3. Atcherson E. Home hemodialysis and the spouse assistant. *J Am Assoc Nephrol Nurses Tech.* 1981 8:29-34

4. Marshall JR, Rice DG, O'Mera M, Shelp WD. Characteristics of couples with poor outcome in dialysis home training. *J Chron Dis.* 1975 28:375-381

5. Streltzer J, Finkelstein F, Feigenbaum H, et al. The spouse's role in home hemodialysis. *Arch Gen Psychiatry.* 1976 33:55-58

Chapter 13

1. Goodkin DA, Pisoni RL, Locatelli F, et al. Hemodialysis vascular access training practices are key to improved access outcomes. *Am J Kidney Dis.* 2010 56(6):1032-42

2. Committee to reduce infection deaths. Accessed on July 22, 2011 at http://www.hospitalinfection.org/protectyourself.shtml

Chapter 14

1. Neumann, ME. 17th annual ranking. *Nephrol News Issues.* 2011 25(8):32-33

Index

Note: 'F' following a page number indicates a figure; 't' indicates a table.

nique, 51; connecting to HD machine, 59; and dental health, 73; infection risk of, 101; and needle removal, 59; overview of, 51–52; and pain management, 63–64, 112, 129; and time commitment, 63; washing before HD, 57. See also access

grief, stages of, 9

H

hair loss, 26

hard water syndrome, 37

health insurance: and dental health, 74; Medigap, 149; and peritoneal dialysis (PD), 99; private, 146–48; and short daily home HD, 111. See also Medicare; Social Security Disability

hearing impaired people, 88

heart health: and anemia, 113, 130; and blood vessel calcification, 30; and electrolytes, 20t; and fistulas, 43; healthy heart vs. heart with LVH, 31; and inflammation, 35; kidney disease's effects on, 14, 25; and nocturnal HD, 134; and poor sleep, 76; and short daily home HD, 118; and standard in-center HD, 64, 68, 77; and water purity, 38

hemodialysis (HD). See dialysis; nocturnal HD; peritoneal dialysis (PD); short daily home HD; standard in-center HD

Hemodoc blog, 161

hemoglobin (Hb), 23, 69, 130, 134–35

heparin: and blood loss, 66t; and dialysis, 36; and hair loss, 26; and menstruation, 29; and peritoneal dialysis (PD) issues, 100

hernia: and automated PD, 85; avoiding, 97; and hospital stays, 157; and peritoneal dialysis (PD), 87, 89–90, 100

HeRO™ graft, 51

home dialysis. See nocturnal HD; peritoneal dialysis (PD); short daily home HD; standard home HD

Home Dialysis Central website, 106, 137, 152, 160

homeostasis: definition of, 16; effects of loss of, 24–31; kidneys' role in creating, 17, 19, 21, 23; lack of, and standard-in center HD, 24, 57, 68, 75; and sexual intimacy, 75; and water levels, 17–19

homocysteine, 22, 118

hormones: antidiuretic hormone (ADH), 17; erythropoietin (EPO), 23, 26; and fertility, 29; leptin, 22; melatonin, 133; parathyroid hormone (PTH), 23, 68, 93, 113, 130; and poor sleep, 76; and sexual intimacy, 26, 75, 97; urodilatin, 17

hospice, 14

hospitalizations: advocates during, 156; as measure of clinic quality, 151, 153; and Medicare coverage, 146; and nocturnal HD, 131, 137; and peritoneal dialy-

sis (PD), 89, 157; preventing infections during, 111, 157–58; protecting access sites during, 53; and short daily home HD, 113; and standard home HD, 82; and standard in-center HD, 70, 120

hospitals: choosing, 156–57; and dialysis clinics, 144; dialysis in, 157; packing for stays in, 158–59. See also surgery

hyperpigmentation, 72

I

immune system, 18, 35, 76, 132, 136, 158

infection: by access types, 101; and Buttonhole technique, 50–51; and catheters, 39–40, 42, 47, 51, 53, 100; and dental visits, 73; and dialyzer reuse, 36; fistulas' low rate of, 43, 47, 51, 53; grafts' rate of, 51; home vs. clinic rates of, 111; and needle insertion, 141; and overweight people, 89; and peritoneal dialysis (PD), 85, 88, 99, 101, 154; and permcath CVCs, 51; and presternal PD catheter, 40; preventing, 49, 51, 58, 97, 157–58; signs of, 49; and swimming, 97; and transfer set, 41; urinary tract, 28

inflammation: and advanced glycation end products (AGEs), 22; and dialysate endotoxins, 37–38; and dialyzer reuse, 36; and joint pain, 29; reducing, 36; results of, 35; and trans fats, 130

Initiating Dialysis Early and Late (IDEAL) study, 32

insurance. See health insurance; Medicare; Social Security Disability

interstitial fluid, 18, 65, 118, 118–19

interstitial spaces, 19

interstitium, 18, 64–65, 134t

intimacy. See sexual intimacy

intracellular spaces, 18–19

ions, 19

iron, 38, 68, 94, 113, 130

irritability, 27

itchy skin, 25

J

joint pain, 29, 89

K

kidney disease: vs. acute illness, 3; causes of, 28; finding meaning in, 8; and life expectancy, 14; number of people with, in U.S., 2; process of, 2; self-management of, 3–4; stages of, 28; statistics on, 150; symptoms of, 24–31; and transplants, 28

kidney doctors. See nephrologists

kidneys, artificial: and itchy skin, 25; used in dialysis, 35–36. See also dialyzers; specific types of dialysis

nutrition. See diet and fluid limits

NxStage System One™, 108, 164

O

obesity. See overweight people

options awareness, 4

osmosis, 19, 38

osteoporosis, 30. See also bone health

overweight people: and peritoneal dialysis (PD), 89; and poor sleep, 76; and presternal PD catheter, 40; and standard in-center HD, 61

Oxalosis and Hyperoxaluria Foundation (OHF), 162

oxygen, 18, 23, 26, 30, 37, 71

P

pain, 63–64, 112, 129. See also joint pain

parathyroid glands, 23. See also hormones

PD. See peritoneal dialysis (PD)

periodic limb movements in sleep (PLMS), 27

peritoneal dialysis (PD): and amputees, 88; and bathing, 39; benefits of, 99–100; biocompatibility of membranes, 35; and blind people, 88; and blood vessel calcification, 30; and body image, 97; and care partners, 139–40; catheters, 39–42; choosing a clinic for, 152–55; choosing type of, 86–87; compared to standard in-center HD, 84; continuous ambulatory PD, 85; convenience of, 5; cycler machines, 85–86, 95–96, 102; and diabetes, 94; dialysate in, 36, 84; diet/fluid limits of, 5, 93; and elderly, 89; encapsulating peritoneal sclerosis (EPS), 101–2; equipment makers, 164; exchanges, 84–85; and exercise, 97; and fertility issues, 98; by hand, 85; and hearing impaired people, 88; and hernias, 89–90, 101; and hospital stays, 157; infection risk of, 101; life expectancy, 78; lifestyle with, 55t, 92–98; low-volume recumbent-only (LVRO), 90; and Medicare coverage, 99; and Medicare payments, 147; medications, 93–94; and membrane failure, 102; Moncrief-Popovich procedure, 40; and overweight people, 89; and parenting, 99; presternal catheter, 40; problems of, 100–102; process of, 84; reasons for exclusion from, 87; sensations during, 92, 102; sepsis risk of, 101; and sexual problems, 97–98; and sleep problems, 98; survival rates, 103; and swimming, 39, 97; time commitment of, 92; training for, 87; and transfer set, 41; and transplants, 99; and travel, 95–97; and weight gain, 102; who can do, 87–90; and work life, 94

peritoneal equilibrium test (PET), 86

peritoneum: and advanced glycation end products (AGEs), 100; definition of, 84; and dialysate, 93; and draining problems, 100; and hernias, 89; and peritoneal dialysis (PD), 35, 39–41, 84; and peritoneal equilibrium test (PET), 86; preventing infection in, 42.

See also peritoneal dialysis (PD)

peritonitis, 42, 89, 99, 101, 157. See also infection

permeability, 34–35, 38

pH levels, 21

phosphate: and blood vessel calcification, 30; description of, 22; effects of, 20t; in enhanced meat products, 67; and itchy skin, 25; and nocturnal HD, 129, 135; and parathyroid hormone (PTH), 23; removal of, 30; and short daily home HD, 119; and sleep problems, 27; and standard in-center HD, 81. See also wastes

phosphate binders, 68, 93–94, 113, 129, 130

phosphorus, 23, 30, 55t, 67, 71, 93, 105t, 113, 129. See also phosphate; wastes

physiologic treatment, 24–25

pica, 26

pills. See medications

pore size. See permeability

positive attitude, 8

potassium: in dialysate, 37; diet limits of, 55t, 67; effects of, 20t; in enhanced meat products, 67; during hospital stays, 157; limits of, on standard in-center HD, 67; and neuropathy, 29; and nocturnal HD, 129; during travel, 117, 131

power of attorney, 14

pregnancy. See fertility

prescriptions. See medications

presternal catheter, 40, 89. See also peritoneal dialysis (PD)

Propublica, 151, 161

protein-bound molecules, 22

proteins, 18, 22, 35, 84

pruritus, 25

pseudoporphyria, 27

Q

quality: of dialysis clinics, 150–55; of life, 120

R

recliners, 148

red blood cells, 23, 26

renal artery stenosis, 28. See also stenosis

renal bone disease, 30

Renal Support Network, 162

renal vitamins, 68, 94, 113, 130

renin, 17

resources, 160–64